HANDBOOK OF VITAMINS AND HORMONES

Roman J. Kutsky, Ph.D.

Associate Professor of Biology
Texas Woman's University
DENTON, TEXAS

VNR **Van Nostrand Reinhold Company**
New York Cincinnati Toronto London Melbourne

Van Nostrand Reinhold Company Regional Offices:
New York   Cincinnati   Chicago   Millbrae   Dallas
Van Nostrand Reinhold Company International Offices:
London   Toronto   Melbourne
Copyright © 1973 by Litton Educational Publishing, Inc.
Library of Congress Catalog Card Number: 70-190499
ISBN: 0-442-24549-1
Manufactured in the United States of America
Published by Van Nostrand Reinhold Company
450 West 33rd Street, New York, N.Y. 10001
Published simultaneously in Canada by Van Nostrand Reinhold Ltd.
15 14 13 12 11 10 9 8 7 6 5 4 3 2 1

Library of Congress Cataloging in Publication Data

Kutsky, Roman J   1922—
    Handbook of vitamins and hormones.

    Bibliography: p.
    1.   Vitamins.   2.   Vitamin therapy.   3.   Hormones.
4.   Hormone therapy.   I.   Title.
RM259.K88   612'.399   70—190499
ISBN 0—442—24549—1

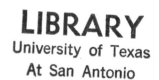

Preface

The properties and modes of action of both the vitamins and the hormones, and their interrelationships to each other as metabolic controlling agents, are easily accessible in this handbook. The book was written to alleviate the continued frustration experienced by many people, including myself, when attempting to obtain unitary, basic information on vitamins and hormones. Although many of the data are separately available, they are so scattered in many compendia, original research papers, and reviews that a small research project on each vitamin and hormone is required before most of the data can be placed in proper context and profitably used. This feeling of dissatisfaction was brought to a head when I recently presented graduate courses in Endocrinology and on Vitamins and Hormones, thus providing the stimulus for this book. Much of the material, and the general format of this volume were generated from lecture notes for the course on Vitamins and Hormones.

It is hoped that this book will be of use to researchers and students in the various fields of life sciences, as well as to physicians, pharmacologists, nurses, and dietitians. Moreover, this book has sufficient content of semitechnical language to make it useful to the educated layman who might need ready information to guide him through the vitamin fads of the day, including rational meal and cooking selections, and to aid in understanding the hormone-related articles in various newspapers and magazines.

I wish to emphasize the fact that conflicting data exist in the various literature sources. The values finally selected, in cases of doubt, were those that could be confirmed by reference to other publications and/or to original literature, where possible. Comments and more recent data are solicited from the readers, especially on individual values and on the format and content of this handbook, as it is my hope to continually improve the usefulness of this volume in future editions.

Many have aided and encouraged me in the preparation of this book. I am grateful to numerous investigators in the fields of nutrition and endocrinology and to my scientific colleagues. In particular I wish to acknowledge the assistance of Dr. Mohamed Aboul-Ela on the sections on plant biosynthesis of vitamins and the aid of Dr. Phyllis Kutsky, my wife, for helpful comments and criticisms and for expediting the final manuscript. My thanks also to Mrs. Bobbie Trietsch for her proficient typing of the manuscript.

I wish to thank the National Academy of Sciences for permission to reproduce the table of RECOMMENDED DAILY DIETARY ALLOWANCES, Seventh Revised Edition, 1968.

Abbreviations

A.A. . . . . amino acid
Absn. . . . . absorption
Acet. . . . . acetone
ACH . . . . acetyl choline
ACTH . . . . . adrenocorticotrop(h)ic
      hormone
ADH . . . . antidiuretic hormone
      (vasopressin)
Ala. . . . . alanine
Aldos. . . . . aldosterone
Alc. . . . . (ethyl) alcohol
Alk. . . . . alkaline
AMP . . . . adenosine monophosphate
$_c$AMP . . . . . . cyclic adenosine mono-
      phosphate
Approx. . . . . approximately
Aq. . . . . aqueous
Arg. . . . . arginine
Asn. . . . . asparagine
Asp. . . . . aspartic acid
ATP . . . . adenosine triphosphate

Benz. . . . . benzene
Bio. . . . . biotin
BMR . . . . basal metabolic rate

CF . . . . citrovorum factor
Chl. . . . . chloroform
CHO . . . . carbohydrate
Chromatog. . . . . chromatograph
CMC, CM cell . . . . . carboxymethyl
      cellulose
CNS . . . . central nervous system
CoA . . . . coenzyme A
Conc. . . . . concentrated
Conv. . . . . converted
CoQ . . . . Coenzyme Q
Cort. . . . . cortisol
CRH . . . . . corticotrop(h)in-releasing
      hormone
Cys. . . . . cysteine

DDT . . . dichloro-diphenyl-trichloro-
      ethane (insecticide)
DEAE . . . . diethylaminoethyl
      (cellulose)
Defic. . . . . deficiency
Dil. . . . . dilute
DOPA . . . . dihydroxyphenylalanine
DPN . diphosphopyridine nucleotide
DNA . . . . deoxyribonucleic acid

vii

Enz. . . . . enzyme

Ep., Epi. . . . . .epinephrine
Equiv. . . . . .equivalent
Esp. . . . . especially
Est. . . . . estradiol
Eth. . . . . ether
Ext. . . . . extract

F.A. . . . . folic acid
FAD . . . .flavin adenine dinucleotide
FMN . . . . . . .flavin mononucleotide
FRH . . . . . . FSH-releasing hormone
FSH . . . .follicle-stimulating hormone
Fluoresc. . . . . fluorescent

GH . . . . . . .growth hormone (STH)
G.I. . . . . gastro-intestinal
Gln. . . . . glutamine
Glu. . . . . .glutamic acid
Gluc(ag). . . . . .glucagon
Gly. . . . . .glycine
GPU . . . . .guinea pig unit
GRH . . . . growth (somatotrop(h)in)
          releasing hormone

HCG . . . . .human chorionic gonado-
          trophin
HGH . . . . . human growth hormone
His. . . . . histidine
HMG . human menopause gonadotro-
          phin (mixture of FSH and LH)
HMP . . . . . .hexose monophosphate
Hyp. R.F., HRH .hypothalamic-releas-
          ing factor (hormone)

Ile. . . . . isoleucine
In. . . . . insulin
Insol. . . . . .insoluble
IRC . . . . ion exchange resin
Irrad. . . . . irradiated
I.U. . . . . international unit
I.V. . . . . intravenous

Leu. . . . . .leucine
LH . . . . luteinizing hormone
LLD . . . . L. lactis Dorner
LRH . . . . . . .LH-releasing hormone
Lys. . . . . .lysine

Max. . . . . .maximum
me. . . . . .methyl
Met. . . . . methionine
Metab. . . . . .metabolism
MIH . . . . . . MSH-inhibiting hormone
Monocl. . . . . monoclinic
MP . . . . .melting point
MRH . . . . . .MSH-releasing hormone
MSH melanocyte-stimulating hormone
MW . . . . molecular weight

NAD(P) . . . nicotinamide adenine di-
          nucleotide (phosphate)
NADPH . . . . .reduced NADP
Nia. . . . . .niacin
NIH . . . National Institutes of Health
Nor., Norepi. . . . . . norepinephrine
NRC . . . .National Research Council

OAA . . . . .oxaloacetic acid
Oxy. . . . . .oxytocin

P.A., Pant. . . . . . pantothenic acid
PBI . . . . protein-bound iodine
Pet. . . . . .petroleum
PGA . . . .pteroyl glutamic acid, folic
          acid
Phe . . . . phenylalanine
pI . . . . .isoelectric point
PIH . . . prolactin-inhibiting hormone
PMSG . . . . . .pregnant mare serum
          gonadotrophin
Ppt. . . . . precipitate
PRH . . . prolactin-releasing hormone
Pro. . . . . .proline
Prog. . . . . progesterone

Prol. . . . . .prolactin
PTH . . . . parathormone

RBC . . . . red blood cell
Relax. . . . . relaxin
RNA . . . . ribonucleic acid
ₘRNA . . . messenger ribonucleic acid

Ser. . . . . .serine
Serot. . . . . serotonin
Sl. . . . . .slightly
Sol. . . . . .soluble
Soln. . . . . solution
Std. . . . . standard
STH . . . . somatotrop(h)in (GH)

T3 . . . . triiodothyronine
T4 . . .tetraiodothyronine (thyroxine)

TCA . . . . tricarboxylic acid (cycle),
            Krebs (cycle)
TCT . . . . thyrocalcitonin
Test., Testos. . . . . testosterone
Thr. . . . . threonine
TPN . . triphosphopyridine nucleotide
         (NADP)
TRH . . . . . .TSH-releasing hormone
Try. . . . . tryptophan
TSH . . . thyroid-stimulating hormone
Tyr. . . . . tyrosine

UDP . . . . uridine diphosphate
USP . . . .*United States Pharmacopeia*
UV . . . . .ultraviolet

Val. . . . . .valine
Vaso. . . . . vasopressin
Vit. . . . . .vitamin

Contents

1
Introduction

With the new discoveries in molecular biology, biochemistry, physiology, and endocrinology, the emphasis in research in life sciences is turning from descriptive biochemistry and electron microscopy to the functional, dynamic aspects of the vital, metabolic processes. In particular, great interest has been generated in the actual controlling agents which accurately blend all the cellular enzyme systems and organelles to produce a living cell, and, from that, a living multicellular organism. It is precisely in this area of control mechanisms that the vitamins and hormones play such a key role, because they are controlling agents.

This book is written primarily from the standpoint of the vitamin and hormone requirements and contents of individuals of the *human* species. It should be understood that requirements and contents differ from species to species, in general becoming simpler as one goes down the evolutionary scale. For the purposes of this book, a *vitamin* is defined as a biologically active, organic compound, a controlling agent essential for an organism's (human's) normal health and growth (its absence causing a deficiency disease or disorder), not synthesized within the organism, available in the diet in small amounts, and carried in the circulatory system in small concentrations to act on target organs or tissues. A *hormone* is defined as a biologically active, organic compound, a controlling agent essential for normal health and growth (its absence causing a deficiency disease or disorder), synthesized within the organism (human being) in ductless glands which release the agent in very small concentrations into the circulatory system to act on the target organs or tissues.

The chief differences between a vitamin and a hormone seem to be the site of biosynthesis, the types of organic compounds present in vitamins as opposed to the hormones, and some of the modes of action. These differences between

1

vitamins and hormones in essential properties are small compared to their similarities and explain why both vitamins and hormones are combined into one book.

In the light of new evidence, it is becoming difficult to differentiate certain vitamins from some hormones. For example, both vitamin D and niacin are synthesized (but in an inadequate amount) in the human, thus conferring on them a hormonal quality. Similarly, the human requirement for the hormone thyroxine can be partially satisfied by a dietary intake of iodine, and some of the steroid hormones are active in a dietary form thus giving them a vitamin quality. Moreover, the fat-soluble vitamins (A, D, E, K) show many similarities in biosynthesis, structure, properties and function to the fat-soluble hormones (steroids). Finally, the same molecule can function as a hormone or as a vitamin depending on the species involved. For example, vitamin C functions as a vitamin in primates because they cannot synthesize it, but it functions as a hormone in rats because they can synthesize it.

We can see that the concept of vitamins and hormones, as defined here, could be extended to all organisms with circulatory systems and would therefore include all vertebrates, many invertebrates, and the higher plants, excepting mainly the lower plants and animals and unicellular organisms. If the definition of circulatory system were to include intracellular circulation, then all living organisms would be included. The concept of vitamin is therefore very much dependent on the species concerned as, if we accept the expanded definition of circulatory system, then the "vitamins" synthesized by unicellular organisms would actually be hormones. Vitamins seem to have arisen very early in the evolution of life as judged by their presence and requirement in some of the most primitive forms of life known today. Hormones, according to our original definition, however, denote a much later period of emergence, becoming prominent mainly with the evolution of the various animals. They, therefore, reflect a shorter evolutionary history. In view of their primitive nature, vitamins would be expected to have, in general, a simpler structure than hormones, and this is indeed the case, with a few exceptions.

As we compare modes of action of vitamins and hormones, we should compare their chemical structures. The vitamins consist of a fat-soluble series and a water-soluble series. The fat-soluble vitamins (A, D, E, K) consist of derivatives of partially cyclized isoprenoid polymers, somewhat similar to the intermediates in cholesterol (steroid) synthesis. These vitamins seem to act by virtue of their lipid solubility in various cell membranes to affect permeability or transport, and by virtue of their chemical groups as redox agents (A, E, K), as coenzymes or enzyme activators (D, K, A), or as enzyme inhibitors (E). The water-soluble vitamins (B_1, B_2, B_6, B_{12}, niacin, pantothenic acid, folic acid, biotin, C) consist, in general, of derivatives or substituted derivatives of sugars (C), pyridine (niacin, B_6), purines and pyrimidines (folic acid, B_2, B_1), amino acid-organic acid complexes (folic acid, biotin, pantothenic acid) and a porphyrin-nucleotide complex (B_{12}). These structurally diverse water-soluble vitamins act as enzyme activators and coenzymes (B_1, B_2, B_6, B_{12}, pantothenic acid, folic acid, biotin, niacin), as redox agents on enzyme reactions (C, B_2, B_{12}, folic acid, niacin) as nuclear agents (folic acid, B_{12}, C, biotin) and probably mitochondrial agents (B_2, C, niacin).

The hormones also include a fat-soluble, steroid series (estradiol, progesterone, aldosterone, testosterone, cortisol) which seems to act (1) by virtue of lipid solubility to stabilize and change permeability of the cell membranes, (2) to regulate enzyme activity and membrane polarization, (3) to regulate redox potential, and (4) to affect RNA transcription in the nucleus (aldosterone, estradiol, testosterone). The water-soluble hormones consist of a protein series (STH, TSH, FSH, LH, Prol.) which seems to act on the cell membrane to stimulate cyclic AMP production with consequent ATP production, and enzyme activation, and to activate certain genes in the nucleus. The peptide series of water-soluble hormones (insulin, glucagon, ACTH, MSH, oxytocin, ADH, PTH, T4, TCT, and relaxin) acts similarly to the proteins and also has an effect on the mitochondria by T4 and PTH. The amine, water-soluble hormone series (epinephrine, norepinephrine) seems to act chiefly by the cyclic AMP mechanism on the membrane, with consequent enzyme activation. The very extensive role of $_c$AMP as an intracellular mediator of hormonal activity is most noteworthy.

It can be seen that the fat-soluble vitamins and hormones act similarly on membranes, on redox potentials, and as enzyme activators, the only difference being in a demonstrated action on the nucleus by the steroids. Comparison of the water-soluble series of hormones with that of the vitamins again shows a basic similarity in action, the vitamins acting as direct enzyme activators and coenzymes, and the hormones acting as indirect activators via cyclic AMP. Both act on the nucleus but differ in that only some of the water-soluble vitamins have redox properties. Again here, the differences between the two water-soluble series of vitamins and hormones lie chiefly in their differing structures and in some of their properties, such as redox regulation and presence of cyclic AMP intermediates.

The subject of vitamin requirements requires comment. There is now sufficient evidence to indicate that the concept of biochemical individuality has much merit. Thus the recommended allowances as stated in this book (NRC Data) should be considered only as average figures, and variations (increase or decrease) of twentyfold or more in individual human requirements may be found, depending on the genetic and physiological state of the individual. Germane to this are the topics of subclinical vitamin deficiencies and megavitamin therapy, i.e., large overdosages of one or more vitamins such as are now being used as treatment of colds and schizophrenia.

The existence of subclinical vitamin deficiencies is extremely difficult to prove without adequate statistical data, but, undoubtedly, if we accept the principle of biochemical individuality, they do exist. In like manner, the use of megavitamins may be helpful to those individuals whose systems for some reason destroy these vitamins rapidly or require these vitamins in large quantity due to their biochemical individuality. However, in view of the fact that accurate data are lacking, megavitamins should be treated and used as drugs with competent medical advice, being wary of possible unexpected individual toxicity.

A perusal of the miscellaneous section for each hormone or vitamin will indicate to the reader the enormous amount of interplay occurring among vitamins and hormones themselves and also with each other. This includes both antagonisms and synergisms occurring simultaneously among various vitamins and hormones. Undoubtedly there exists an optimal set of levels for each vitamin and hormone which, presumably, is that which has been found in "normal" human values. But maximum optimization of levels at "normal" human values has not been proven experimentally; perhaps the human system could run more efficiently at a different set of values. More research is needed to determine this. In any case, optimum amounts and ratios of all vitamins and hormones are important to get full benefits of these agents.

Lack of space and time has precluded extensive mention of the trace elements and mineral cofactors required for functioning of most coenzyme systems as well as some hormones, e.g., magnesium, iron, copper, iodine, selenium, cobalt, etc. These trace elements should be present in correct amounts and ratios in any balanced diet containing adequate vitamins.

In relation to requirements, the subject of undiscovered or unaccepted vitamins and hormones should be mentioned. This book has included only those vitamins and hormones with widespread acceptance. In addition to the 13 vitamins listed here, there are at least another 13 compounds with various acceptabilities as vitamins, plus possibly other vitamins still undiscovered. In relationship to individual requirements, this means that taken together with the facts of mutual interdependence of vitamins as mentioned above, it would still be advisable to rely for one's vitamin requirement chiefly on rich natural sources in the diet, since these would most likely contain the undiscovered vitamins. However, in view of the possible extreme losses of vitamin potency even in our richest dietary sources caused by our present methods of processing, storing, and cooking of food, it would be advisable to consider vitamin supplementation of certain vitamins, especially if one's diet has not been carefully planned.

As far as the hormones are concerned, at least another 23 compounds, in addition to the 23 listed here, are known with various degrees of acceptance as true hormones. No doubt many more remain to be discovered. This book has not listed the insect or plant hormones, because the human requirements and levels are being stressed.

2
Presentation
of Data

This book will serve as a ready reference to four major groups of readers, inasmuch as the data for each vitamin and hormone are presented in several separate sections, as follows: "General Information" and "Miscellaneous Information" for the general reader and all other groups; "Medical and Biological Role" mainly for the biologists, physicians, nurses, and pharmacologists; "Chemical Properties" and "Metabolic Properties" for the biochemists and physiologists; and "Nutritional Role" for dietitians and nutritionists. However, it is hoped that parts of all sections will be useful to all the groups. Insofar as possible, the format is similar for both hormones and vitamins for ease of reference. A list of abbreviations is given at the beginning of the book.

The specific vitamins and hormones chosen for coverage in this book are those that have the widest acceptance by the various workers in both fields. Only the most active of the steroid hormones in each category of mineralocorticoids, glucocorticoids, and sex hormones in the human is being covered (out of the 40 plus already discovered).

Chapters on Vitamins and Hormones

General Information Section

"Active analogs and related compounds" includes vitamers, isotels, etc.

"Antagonists" and "Synergists" may be the same chemical species but in different concentrations. Interaction at the target site is used as a criterion of antagonism or synergism.

"Sources for Species" (Essentiality) indicates degree of requirement for various species including man. Endogenous = made within organism. Exogenous sources include intestinal bacteria.

Chemical Properties Section

"Reactions" refers to those carried out with standard laboratory conditions and reagents and not under extreme conditions, unless otherwise noted. i.e., heat $\leqslant 100°C$, weak acids or alkalies, reactivity with water, atmospheric or mild oxidation agents, mild reducing agents, bright daylight.

Isolation method gives a typical procedure now in use.

Medical and Biological (Nutritional) Section

This provides, in general, clinical information. Contents of vitamins are per 100 g. edible portion

Antigenicity is defined as the ability to act as an antigen creating an immune response when administered to an organism. Specificity is here defined as the degree of restriction of biological activity to a certain species.

Metabolic Role Section

"Enzyme Reactions" lists enzyme systems affected by the vitamin or hormone, organ location, and effects on enzymes, where known.

"Mode of Action" subdivides functions on both a cellular basis (anabolic, catabolic, etc.) and an organismal basis. Anabolic denotes synthetic processes; catabolic denotes degredative reactions and includes most energy yielding reactions.

Miscellaneous Information Section

"Relationships to other Vitamins, Hormones" attempts to indicate the mutual involvement of both vitamins and hormones in most actions of both groups either together or within the group.

"Unusual Features" includes various chemical, biological, and pharmacological features that could not be listed elsewhere.

"Possible Relationships" attempts to draw a parallel between the action of vitamin or a hormone and its deficiency symptoms.

The tables following Chapter 38 list in tabular fashion some of the data already presented and some new data in an attempt to indicate fundamental similarities and dissimilarities in structure and function of both vitamins and hormones.

References are presented in numbered form at the end of the book, and are subdivided into three categories: General; Specific: Vitamins; and Specific: Hormones. An effort has been made to cite only the latest available handbooks, compendia, journal references, and texts.

3
Vitamin A

GENERAL INFORMATION

1. **Synonyms:** Retinol, axerophthol, biosterol, vitamin A_1, anti-xerophthalmic vitamin, anti-infective vitamin

2. **History**
   - 1912—Hopkins reported factor in milk needed for growth of rats
   - 1913—Osborne and Mendel demonstrated milk factor is fat soluble; present in other fats also
   - 1913-15—McCollum and Davis identified milk factor (fat-soluble A) in butter, egg yolk
   - 1917—McCollum and Simmonds found xerophthalmia in rats due to lack of fat-soluble A
   - 1920—Drummond renamed fat-soluble A, vit. A
   - 1930—Moore determined carotene a precursor for vit. A
   - 1930-37—Karrer *et al.* isolated and synthesized vit. A
   - 1935—Wald reported visual purple in retina a complex of protein and vit. A

3. **Physiological Forms**
   Retinol (vit. A_1) and esters
   3-Dehydroretinol (vit. A_2) and esters
   Retinal (retinene, vit. A aldehyde), 3-dehydroretinal (retinine-2)
   Retinoic acid
   Neovitamin A
   Neo-b-vit. A_1

7

4. **Active Analogs and Related Compounds:** α, β, γ-carotene, neo-β-carotene B, cryptoxanthine, myxoxanthine, torularhodin, aphanicin, echinenone

5. **Inactive Analogs and Related Compounds:**   Kitol, xanthophyll, lycopene

6. **Antagonists:**   Sodium benzoate, bromobenzene, citral, oxidized derivatives of vit. A, thyroxine (large concentrations), estrogens, vitamin E (membrane permeability)

7. **Synergists:**   Vitamins B_2, B_{12}, C, E, thyroxine, testosterone, MSH, STH

8. **Physiological Functions:**   Growth, production of visual purple, maintenance of skin and epithelial cells, resistance to infection, gluconeogenesis, mucopolysaccharide synthesis, bone development, maintenance of myelin and membranes, maintenance of color and peripheral vision, maintenance of adrenal cortex and steroid hormone synthesis

9. **Deficiency Diseases, Disorders:**   Xerophthalmia, nyctalopia, hemeralopia, keratomalacia, hyperkeratosis

10. **Sources for Species Requiring It**
    Required by many animal species
    Exogenous sources—All vertebrates and some invertebrates convert plant dietary carotenoids in gut to vit. A_1, which is absorbed
    Endogenous sources—None reported

CHEMISTRY

1. **Structure**

Vitamin A_1, $C_{20}H_{30}O$

β-ionone

2. **Reactions**

Heat—Labile (isomerizes)
Acid—Labile (isomerizes)
Alkali—Stable
Water—Insol.

Oxidation—Labile (isomerizes)
Reduction—Stable
Light—Labile (isomerizes) (UV
  inactivates)

3. **Properties**

Appearance—Yellow oil
MW—286.4
MP—62-64°C
Crystal Form—Prisms
Salts, Esters—Acetate palmi-
  tate
Important Groups for activity
  β-ionone ring
  trans-methyl
  Alcoholic hydroxyl

Solubility
  H_2O—Insol.
  Acet., Alc.—Sol.
  Chl., Eth.—Sol.
Absn. Max.—325-328 mμ
Chemical Nature—Unsaturated alc.
$\alpha_D = 0$ (inactive)

4. **Commercial Production**

Chemical—Extraction of fish liver
Synthetic—From citral or β-ionone

5. **Isolation**

Sources—Fish liver oils
Method—Saponification in alcoholic KOH. Extract with ether, crystallize

6. **Determination**

Bioassay—Growth rate of rats
Physicochemical—Spectrophotometric determination of blue color on
    reacting with antimony trichloride or trifluoracetic acid

DISTRIBUTION AND SOURCES

1. **Occurrence**

Plants
    Fruit—Provitamin carotenoids—apricots, yellow melons, peaches,
      prunes
    Vegetables—Provitamin carotenoids—beet greens, broccoli greens,
      carrots, endive, kale, lettuce, mint, mustard, parsley, pumpkins,
      spinach, sweet potatoes, turnip greens, cress
    Nuts—Provitamin carotenoids—in small quantity in most nuts

Animals:

Vitamin A in all vertebrates, and carotenoids in certain invertebrates (crustacea) (A_2 especially in fresh-water fish)

Location: Liver, heart, lungs, fat, adrenals, retina, kidney, milk, blood plasma, egg

Provitamin carotenoids found in many animals depending on diet

Hen's egg carotenoid mainly xanthophyll (inactive analog)

Microorganisms: Provitamin carotenoids in algae, fungi, bacteria. No intestinal synthesis of vit. A

2. **Dietary Sources:**   (Vit. A and Procarotenoids)

High: 10,000–76,000 I.U./100 g

Liver (beef, pig, sheep, calf, chicken)

Liver oil (cod, halibut, salmon, shark, sperm whale)

Carrots, mint, kohlrabi, parsley, spinach, turnip greens, dandelion greens, palm oil

Medium: 1000-10,000 I.U./100 g

Butter, cheese (except cottage), egg yolk, margarine, dried milk, cream

White fish, eel

Kidneys (beef, pig, sheep), liver (pork)

Mangoes, apricots, yellow melons, peaches, cherries (sour), nectarines

Beet greens, broccoli, endive, kale, mustard, pumpkin, sweet potatoes, watercress, tomatoes, leek greens, chicory, chives, collards, fennel, butterhead and romaine lettuce, squash (acorn, butternut, hubbard), chard

Low: 100-1000 I.U./100 g

Milk

Herring, salmon, oyster, carp, clams, sardines

Grapes, bananas, berries (black-, goose-, rasp-, boysen-, logan-, blue-), sweet cherries, olives, oranges, avocados, prunes, kumquats, pineapples, plums, rhubarb, tangerines, red currants

Summer and zucchini squash, asparagus, beans (except kidney), brussel sprouts, cabbages, leeks, peas, artichokes, corn, cucumbers, lentils (dry), peppers, lettuce, celery, cowpeas, rutabagas, okra

Hazelnuts, peanuts, black walnuts, cashew, pecans, pistachios

MEDICAL AND NUTRITIONAL ROLE

1. **Units:**   1 I.U. = 0.344 μg vit. A acetate = 0.3 μg retinol

2. **Normal Blood Levels:**   100-300 I.U./100 ml serum

3. **Recommended Allowances**
   Children—2000-3500 I.U./day
   Adults—5000 I.U./day
   Special—Pregnancy—6000 I.U./day, Lactation—8000 I.U./day

4. **Administration**
   Injection—Parenteral
   Topical—No data
   Oral—Preferred route

5. **Factors Affecting Availability**
   Decrease
   Liver damage
   Impaired intestinal conversion of carotenes
   Impaired absorption (low bile)
   Food preparation (cooking and frying—heat oxidation)
   Presence of antagonists
   Illness—increased destruction and excretion
   Increase
   Storage in body (liver)
   Intestinal conversion of carotenes—T4, insulin increase
   Absorption aids—bile, fat
   Dietary protein—mobilizes Vit. A from storage in liver

6. **Deficiency Symptoms**
   General
   Retarded growth
   Night blindness (nyctalopia)—degeneration of retina
   Hyperkeratinization of epithelial tissues—
   Degenerative changes in eye epithelium (xerophthalmia, hemeralopia)
   Atrophy of odontoblasts
   Lab animals
   Poor bone and tooth development
   Resorption of fetus, atrophy of germinal epithelium
   Urolithiasis—urinary calculi

7. **Effects of Overdose**
   100,000 units/day (man)—generally toxic
   Irritability, nerve lesions
   Fatigue, insomnia, painful bones and joints
   Exophthalmia
   Mucous cell formation in keratinized membranes

Abnormal bone growth
Loss of hair, jaundice, itchy skin, anorexia
Decreased clotting time
Elevated serum alkaline phosphatase

METABOLIC ROLE

1. Biosynthesis
Precursors
Animals—Carotenoid conversion
(except rat, pig, sheep, carnivores, some invertebrates and human infants)—cannot convert
α, β, γ-carotenes, cryptoxanthin, myxoxanthin, torularhodin
Plants—Cholesterol pathways—acetate, etc., aphanicin, echinenone
Intermediates
Plants—Mevalonic acid, squalene

2. Production: Species and sites
Plants (carotenoids)
Higher plants—Green leaves, yellow vegetables and fruits
Some algae, fungi, bacteria—carotenoids
Animals
Most vertebrates (except rat, pig, sheep)
Conversion of carotenoids to vit. A in intestinal wall
Some invertebrates also convert

3. Storage Sites: Liver, kidney (rat, cat)

4. Blood Carriers
α_1 and α_2-globulins, β-lipoproteins (carotenoids)
Retinol esters via lymphatics (esp. palmitate)
chylomicrons in lymphatics (retinol esters)

5. Half-life: Weeks or months

6. Target Tissues: Retina, skin, bone, liver, adrenals, germinal epithelium

7. Reactions

Coenzyme forms—Neo-b-vit. A_1, retinoic acid

Organ	Enzyme System	Effect
Adrenal cortex	Hydroxylating—deoxycorticosterone → corticosterone	Activated
Liver	Sulfurylases—ATP + SO_4 = phospho-adenosinephosphosulfate	Activated
Intestine	Esterases—Vitamin A ester → vit. A + fatty acid	Activated
Intestine	Synthetases—Vit. A + Fatty acid → vit. A ester	Activated
Liver	Dehydrogenases—neo-b-vit. A_1 → retinene, retinal → retinoic acid	Activated
Retina	Isomerases—*trans*-retinene → *cis*-retinene (inactive)	Activated
Liver	Hydrolases—Acid phosphatase, β-glucuronidase, cathepsin, etc., in lysosomes on hyper- or hypo-vitaminosis A	Released

8. Mode of Action

Cellular

Anabolic—Synthesis of mucopolysaccharides via "active" sulfate. Synthesis of corticosterone

Catabolic—No data

Other—Precursor of retinene in retina—forms visual pigments. Maintains stability of lysosomes + cell membranes

Organismal

Maintenance of visual sense organs

Maintains reproductive systems

Maintains glucocorticoid production in adrenals

Maintains mucous membranes

Regulates cartilage for bone development

9. Catabolism

Intermediates—Retinoic acid

Excretion products

Urine—Vitamin A (only in disease)

fatty acid, small soluble molecules

Breath—CO_2

MISCELLANEOUS

1. Relationship to Other Vitamins

Vitamin C—Plasma vit. C levels drop on depletion of vit. A, occurrence and action of vits. A and C coincide often

Vitamin D—Occurs naturally with vit. A in animal liver oils. Toxic overdose effects reduced by vit. A

Niacin—Involved with DPN + vit. A in activity of retinene reductase.

Vitamin E—Decreases serum cholesterol in rabbit when given with vit. A

Protects vit. A from oxidation

Similarity of structure to vitamin A

Antagonistic to vit. A in maintaining membrane permeability

Pantothenic acid—Promotes synthesis of vit. A in plants

2. Relationship to Hormones

Thyroxine—Stimulates intestinal conversion of carotene to vit. A

Increases vit. A storage in liver

Antagonizes decreased basal metabolism caused by vit. A

Increases use of vit. A

Insulin—Stimulates intestinal conversion of carotene to vit. A

STH—A synergist in growth

Cortisol, Aldosterone, Testosterone, Progesterone—Decreased on vit. A depletion (chemical adrenalectomy). Production of deoxycortico-sterone and other steroids stimulated by vit. A

Estradiol—Antagonistic to vit. A peripherally

MSH—Decreases dark adaptation time—synergistic to vit. A

3. Unusual Features

Decreases serum cholesterol in large quantity administration (chicks)

Dietary protein required to mobilize liver reserves of vit. A

Decreased in tumors

Coenzyme Q_{10} accumulates in A-deficient rat liver

Ubichromenol-50 accumulation in A-deficient rat liver

Retinoic acid functions as vit. A except for visual and reproductive functions

Anti-infection properties and anti-allergic properties

Decreases basal metabolism

Detoxification of poisons in the liver aided by vit. A

Involved in triose $\rightarrow$ glucose conversions

4. **Possible Relationships of Deficiency Symptoms to Metabolic Action**

   Growth Retardation—Effects on steroid synthesis, bone growth, and membrane structure, and development of epithelial tissues

   Keratinization—Effects on membranes and mucopolysaccharide biosynthesis

   Bone development—Formation of chondroitin sulfate in cartilage

   Reproductive failure—Effects on membranes and steroid hormones

   Visual defects—Absence of retinene precursors

4
Vitamin D

GENERAL INFORMATION

1. **Synonyms:** Antirachitic vitamin, vitamin D_3, rachitamin, rachitasterol, cholecalciferol, activated 7-dehydrocholesterol

2. **History**
   1918—Mellanby produced experimental rickets in dogs
   1919—Huldschinsky ameliorated rachitic symptoms in children with ultraviolet irradiation
   1922—Hess showed liver oils contain same antirachitic factor as sunlight
   1922—McCollum increased calcium deposition in rachitic rats with cod liver oil factor
   1924—Steenbook and Hess demonstrated irradiated foods have antirachitic properties
   1925—McCollum named antirachitic factor vit. D.
   1931—Angus isolated crystalline vit. D (calciferol)
   1936—Windaus isolated vit. D_3 (activated 7-dehydrocholesterol)

3. **Physiological Forms:** Vitamin D_2 (calciferol, ergocalciferol), vit. D_3 (cholecalciferol), phosphate esters of D_2, D_3, 25-hydroxycholecalciferol, 1,25-dihydroxycholecalciferol, 5,25-dihydroxycholecalciferol

4. **Active Analogs and Related Compounds:** Irrad. [22-dihydroergosterol (vit. D_4) 2-dehydrostigmasterol (vit. D_6), 7-dehydrositosterol (vit. D_5)]. Dihydrotachysterol

16

5. **Inactive Analogs and Related Compounds:**   Lumisterol, tachysterol, ergosterol, 7-dehydrocholesterol

6. **Antagonists:**   Toxisterol, phytin, phlorizin, cortisone, cortisol, thyrocalcitonin, PTH

7. **Synergists:**   Niacin, PTH, STH

8. **Physiological Functions:**   Normal growth (via bone growth), Ca and P absorption from intestine, antirachitic, increases tubular P reabsorption, increases citrate blood levels, maintains and activates alkaline phosphatase in bone, and maintains serum calcium and phosphorus levels

9. **Deficiency Diseases, Disorders:**   Rickets, osteomalacia, hypoparathyroidism

10. **Sources for Species Requiring It:**   Required by vertebrates
    Exogenous sources—Infant vertebrates and deficient adult vertebrates
    Endogenous sources—Vertebrates (synthesized in skin under UV irrad.)

CHEMISTRY

1. **Structure**

Vitamin D$_3$,
C$_{27}$H$_{44}$O

2. **Reactions**

Heat—Stable	Oxidation—Unstable
Acid—Stable	Reduction—Stable
Alkali—Stable	Light—Unstable
Water—Insol.	

3. Properties

Appearance—White powder

MW—384.65

MP—84-85°C

Form—Fine needles

Salts, Esters

  Palmitate, 3,5-dinitrobenzoate

Important Groups for Activity

  C_{10}–C_{18} Methylene

  Alcoholic—OH

Solubility

  H_2O—Insol.

  Acet., Alc.—Sol.

  Benz., Chl., Eth.—Sol.

Absn. Max.—265 mμ

Chemical Nature—Sterol, alc.

α_D^{20} = +102.5° (alc.)

4. Commercial Production

Irradiation of ergosterol, 7-dehydrocholesterol

Extraction of fish liver oils

5. Isolation

Sources—Liver oil, irradiated yeast

Method—Saponify oil, remove vit. A and sterols by partitioning solvents, and adsorption chromatography, remove inactive sterols with digitonin, crystallize as 3,5-dinitrobenzoate ester, saponify, recrystallize

6. Determination

Bioassay—Antirachitic test on rats

Physicochemical—Reaction with antimony trichloride

DISTRIBUTION AND SOURCES

1. Occurrence

Plants

  Fruit—None

  Vegetables—Grain and vegetable oils (provitamins)

  Nuts—None

Animals: Tuna, halibut, cod liver oils

  Egg yolk, milk (irrad.), bones, intestine, blood, brain, skin, spleen, fish liver

  Shrimp, mollusks

Microorganisms: Yeast, algae, bacteria (provitamins)

2. **Dietary Sources**
    High: $1000\text{-}25 \times 10^6$ I.U./100 g
        Liver oils (bonito, tuna, lingcod, sea bass, swordfish, halibut, herring, cod, sablefish, soupfin shark)
    Medium: 100-1000 I.U./100 g
        Egg yolk, margarine, lard, herring, salmon, mackerel, pilchards, sardines, shrimp, tuna, kippers
    Low: 10-100 I.U./100 g
        Grain and vegetable oils
        Cod roe, halibut
        Butter, cream, eggs, cheeses, milk (vit. D or irrad.)
        Liver (calf, pork, lamb, beef)
        Veal, horse meat, beef

MEDICAL AND NUTRITIONAL ROLE

1. **Units:**   1 U.S.P. = 1 I.U. = 0.025 μg vit. D_3

2. **Normal Blood Levels:**   2.75 μg/100 ml (serum); 66-165 I.U./100 ml (serum)

3. **Recommended Allowances**
    Children—400 I.U./day
    Adults—None in equatorial zones; 400 I.U./day in temperate zones (available in normal diet)
    Special—Pregnancy, 400 I.U./day; lactation, 400 I.U./day; senility, night workers, miners, northern people

4. **Administration**
    Injection—Subcutaneous, intraperitoneal, intramuscular (D_3 esters)
    Topical—Absorbed through skin
    Oral—Preferred route

5. **Factors Affecting Availability**
    Decrease
        Liver damage
        Presence of antagonists
        Presence of phytin in gut
        Low bile salts in gut

High pH in gut
Destruction by intestinal flora
Excretion in feces
Increase
Storage in liver, skin
Absorption aids—bile salts
Long acting feature (slow destruction)
Decrease in pH of lower intestine
Irradiation by UV

6. Deficiency Symptoms
In young or experimental animals, including man
Retarded growth—Rickets
Malformation of long bones—Rickets
Skeletal malformation
Demineralization of bone
Decreased blood calcium and phosphorus
Increased serum alkaline phosphatase

7. Effects of Overdose (Man)—Generally toxic
4000 (or more) I.U./day
Anorexia, nausea, thirst, diarrhea
Polyuria, muscular weakness, joint pains
Increased serum calcium—calcification of soft tissues (arteries, muscle)
Resorption of bone
Arterial lesions and kidney injury (rats)

METABOLIC ROLE

1. Biosynthesis
Precursors—Cholesterol (skin—UV) animals; ergosterol (algae, yeast-UV)
    plants
Intermediates—Pre-ergocalciferol, tachysterol, 7-dehydrocholesterol

2. Production: Species and Site
Plants—Leaves, seeds, shoots (provitamins)
Fungi—Various
Bacteria—Various, but no intestinal synthesis
Animals—Skin

3. Storage Sites: Animals—Liver, skin

4. **Blood Carriers:**   Lipoproteins $(\alpha + \beta)$

5. **Half-life:**   Long acting (days, weeks)

6. **Target Tissues:**   Kidney, bone, intestine, liver

7. **Reactions**
   Reactive form—25-Hydroxycholecalciferol and metabolites
   Coenzyme forms—Phosphorylated vit. D

Organ	Enzyme System	Effect
Intestine	Phytase	Activated
Serum	Alk. phosphatase—Organic phosphate (serum) → inorganic phosphate	Activated
Liver	Phosphorylase—Glycogen → glucose-1-phosphate	Activated

8. **Mode of Action**
   Cellular
       Anabolic—Increases protein synthesis in intestinal cells
       Catabolic
           Depresses protein synthesis except in intestinal cells
       Other
           Decreases citrate oxidation
           Increases release of calcium by mitochondria
           Activates active transport of calcium by intestinal cells
           Repair of mitochondrial membrane
           Regulates phosphorus metabolism
   Organismal
       Promotes normal bone calcification
       Increases formation of osteoclasts and capillaries in cartilage—Increases cartilage degeneration in normal bone calcification
       Regulates phosphorus and calcium metabolism—increases calcium absorption by intestine—Maintains normal serum calcium and phosphorus levels
       Mobilizes phosphorus from soft tissues
       Mobilizes calcium from bone in hypocalcemia (with PTH)
       Converts organic phosphates to inorganic phosphates
       Catabolic

9. **Catabolism**
   Intermediates—Similar to cholesterol conversion products: bile acids and
        steroid hormones
   Excretion products
      No vit. D in urine (human)
      Animals—Excess vit. D into feces
      Humans—70% of ingested vit. D in feces as fecal sterols

MISCELLANEOUS

1. **Relationship to Other Vitamins**
   Vitamin A—
      Reduces toxic effects of vit. D
      Occurs naturally with vit. D in many fish oils
   Vitamin B_1 —Increases tolerance of vit. D

2. **Relationship to Hormones**
   Parathormone—activity intensified by vit. D; deficiency of vit. D
        stimulates parathyroid
   Cortisone—Antagonizes effect of vit. D on citrate metabolism
   STH—A synergist in growth

3. **Unusual Features**
   Has hormonal qualities due to internal synthesis
   Vitamin D_2 little activity for chickens—species differ in response.
   May play role in aging calcification phenomena, especially in skin
   Can mimic rickets with high calcium low phosphorus diet
   Can mimic osteomalacia with low calcium high phosphorus diet
   Absorbed through skin
   Activates transport of heavy metals by intestinal cells
   Ample available for adults from most diets and skin synthesis
   Long acting, stored
   Furred and feathered animals obtain vit. D in grooming and licking
   Fish thought to obtain vit. D from marine invertebrates
   Useful in lead poisoning treatment

4. **Possible Relationships of Deficiency Symptoms to Metabolic Action**
   Decreased growth—Retarded calcification and bone growth
   Increased alkaline phosphatase—Attempt by organism to increase
        inorganic phosphate
   Osteomalacia—Demineralization of bone, (e.g. in pregnancy)
   Skeletal malformation—Retarded calcification

5
Vitamin E

GENERAL INFORMATION

1. **Synonyms:** α-Tocopherol, antisterility vitamin, 5,7,8,-trimethyltocol, Epsilan, Ephynal, Tokopharm, factor X

2. **History**
    1922—Evans and Bishop reported dietary factor "X" needed for normal rat reproduction
    1922—Matill found dietary factor "X" in yeast or lettuce
    1923—Evans *et al.* found factor "X" in alfalfa, wheat, oats, meat, butterfat
    1924—Sure named factor "X" vit. E.
    1936—Evans *et al.* demonstrated vit. E belongs to tocopherol family of compounds—isolated several active tocopherols—vit. E (α-tocopherol) most active of tocopherols
    1938—Fernholz determined structure of vit. E
    1938—Karrer synthesized vit. E
    1956—Green discovered eighth tocopherol

3. **Physiological Forms**
    d-α-tocopherol, tocopheronolactone, and their phosphate esters

4. **Active Analogs and Related Compounds**
    dl-α-Tocopherol, l-α-tocopherol, esters (succinate, acetate, phosphate), β, ζ_1, ζ_2-tocopherols

23

5. **Inactive Analogs and Related Compounds:** δ, ϵ, η-tocopherols

6. **Antagonists:** α-tocopherol quinone, oxidants, cod liver oil, thyroxine

7. **Synergists:**   Vitamins A, B_6, B_{12}, C, K, folic acid, estradiol, testosterone, STH

8. **Physiological Functions**
   Biological antioxidant
   Normal growth maintenance
   Protects unsaturated fatty acids and membrane structures
   Aids intestinal absorption of unsaturated fatty acids
   Maintains normal muscle metabolism
   Maintains integrity of vascular system and central nervous system
   Detoxifying agent
   Maintenance of kidney tubules, lungs, genital structures, liver and RBC
       membranes

9. **Deficiency Diseases and Disorders**
   Laboratory animals—Degeneration of reproductive tissues, muscular
       dystrophy, encephalomalacia, liver necrosis
   Man—Skin collagenosis, red cell hemolysis, xanthomatosis, cirrhosis of
       gall bladder, steatorrhea, creatinuria

10. **Sources for Species Requiring It**
    Required by most organisms
        Exogenous sources—Man and higher vertebrates, protozoa, some
            microorganisms
        Endogenous sources—Plants, some microorganisms

CHEMISTRY

1. **Structure**

Vitamin E, $C_{29}H_{50}O_2$

2. **Reactions**

Heat—Labile	Oxidation—Labile
Acid—Stable	Reduction—Stable
Alkali—Labile	Light—Labile (esp. UV)
Water—Insol.	

3. **Properties**

Appearance—Yellow oil   Solubility
MW—430.7 H_2O—Insol.
MP—2.5-3.5°C   Acet., Alc.—Sol.
Crystal Form—No data   Benz., Chl., Eth.—Sol.
Salts, Esters—Succinate,   Absn. Max.—292 mμ (alc.)
  acetate, phosphate   Chemical Nature: Aromatic quinoid,
Important Groups for activity   alc.
  Hydroxyl (alcoholic) $\alpha_D^{25} = +0.32°$ (alc.)

4. **Commercial Production:** Molecular distillation from vegetable oils

5. **Isolation**

  Sources—Wheat germ oil, soybean oil, rice oil
  Method
    Saponify oil with methanolic KOH
    Nonsaponifiable fraction has vit. E, dissolve in ether
    Remove sterols with digitonin precipitation
    Remove xanthophylls with methanol extraction
    Convert tocopherols to allophanate esters with HCN
    Crystallize allophanates, hydrolyze, extract vit. E with ether

6. **Determination**

  Bioassay
    Rats—Prevent fetal resorption and RBC hemolysis
    Chick—Liver storage
  Physicochemical—Colorimetric 2-dimensional paper chromatography

DISTRIBUTION AND SOURCES

1. **Occurrence**

  Plants
    Fruit—Apples, olives

Vegetables—Legumes, lettuce, spinach, corn, soybean (oil), mustard, cauliflower, green peppers, turnip greens, kale, kohlrabi, sweet potatoes

Nuts and Seeds—Coconuts, peanuts, palm (oil), cottonseed

Grains—Cereals, oils (rice, wheat) oats, brown rice, wheat germ, barley, rye

Animals

Birds—Eggs

Mammals—Liver, fat, muscle, milk, pituitary, adrenals, testes

Microorganisms: Yeast

2. Dietary Sources

High: 50-300 mg/100 g

Oil (cottonseed, corn, soybean, safflower, wheat germ)

Margarine

Medium: 5-50 mg/100 g

Oils (coconut, peanut, olive)

Wheat germ, apple seeds, alfalfa, barley, dry soybeans, peanuts

Chocolate, rose hips, yeast

Cabbage, spinach, asparagus

Low: 0.5-5 mg/100 g

Brussel sprouts, carrots, parsnips, mustard, corn, brown rice, lettuce, cauliflower, peas, sweet potatoes, turnip greens, kale, kohlrabi, green peppers

Bacon, beef, lamb, pork, veal, beef liver

Eggs, butter, cheese

Whole wheat flour, dried navy beans, corn meal, oatmeal, coconut, rye, oats, wheat

Blackberries, pears, apples, olives

MEDICAL AND NUTRITIONAL ROLE

1. Units:

1 mg d-α-tocopherol = 1.49 I.U.

1 mg dl-α-tocopherol acetate = 1 I.U.

2. Normal Blood Levels (Man):   1.11 mg/100 ml (serum)

3. Recommended Allowances

Children—10-15 I.U./day

Adults—25 I.U./day (females); 30 I.U./day (males)

Special—Related to unsaturated fatty acid intake; increased requirements in pregnancy and lactation, detoxification, aging, stress

4. **Administration**
    Injection—No data
    Topical—No data
    Oral—Preferred route

5. **Factors Affecting Availability**
    Decrease
       Presence of antagonists
       Mineral oil ingestion
       Presence of vit. E oxidation products
       Occurrence with other less active analogues
       Excretion in feces
       Impaired fat absorption
       Chemical binding in foods
       Increased destruction (stress)
       Cooking losses—Heat and O_2 labile
       Losses in frozen storage, steatorrhea, variability of natural sources
    Increase
       Storage in (adipose and muscle) tissue
       Esterification increases stability
       Use of unprocessed fresh food sources
       Absorption aids—Bile salts

6. **Deficiency Symptoms**
    General
       RBC hemolysis
       Creatinuria
       Xanthomatosis and cirrhosis of gall bladder
       Steatorrhea (young)
       Cystic fibrosis of pancreas (young)
       Poorly developed muscles
    Muscular dystrophy (rats, dogs, monkeys, chickens)
    Myocardial degeneration (dogs, rabbits)
    Resorption of fetus, degeneration of germ epithelium, disturbance of estrus cycle (rats)
    Hepatic necrosis (rats)
    Encephalomalacia (chickens)
    Vascular degeneration (chickens)

7. Effects of Overdose: Possible increase in blood pressure

METABOLIC ROLE

1. **Biosynthesis**
   Precursors—Mevalonic acid—Side chain (?); phenylalanine—ring (?)
   Intermediates—Tocotrienol

2. **Production:**   Species and Sites
   Plants—Nuts, seeds, cereal germ, green leaves, legumes
   Fungi—Yeast
   Bacteria—Various

3. **Storage Sites**
   Muscle—Small amounts
   Adipose tissues—Small amounts

4. **Blood Carriers:**   Lipoproteins

5. **Half-life:**   60-70% of daily dose ingested is excreted in feces

6. **Target Tissues:**   Kidneys, genital organs, muscles, liver, lungs, bone marrow

7. **Reactions**

Organ	Enzyme System
Muscle	Dehydrogenase Xanthine oxidase Isocitric dehydrogenase
Muscle	Protease—Cathepsin
Muscle	Phosphatase Ribonuclease Nucleotidase
Muscle	Glycosidase—glucuronidase
Muscle	Miscellaneous Creatine kinase Cytochrome c reductase

8. Mode of Action

Cellular

Anabolic—Maintains protein synthesis by prevention of formation of enzyme-toxic peroxides from unsaturated fatty acid

Catabolic—Participates in oxidation-reduction reactions via CoQ and respiratory enzyme systems

Other—Protects unsaturated fatty acids against oxidation; maintains structure of cellular, mitochondrial, microsomal, and lysosomal membranes

Organismal

Anabolic—increases N retention

Maintains kidney tubules and genital organs

Maintains muscle cell membranes

9. Catabolism

Intermediates—tocopheryl-*p*-quinone

Excretion products

Breath—CO_2

Urine—Water soluble degradation products, tocopheronic acid glucuronate, tocopheronolactone glucuronate

MISCELLANEOUS

1. Relationship to Other Vitamins

Vitamin C—Reduces oxidized vit. E back to vit. E in rats

Decreased synthesis of vit. C in vit. E deficient animals

Vitamin A—Conserved by vit. E in chick; protected against oxidation by vit. E; synergizes with vit. E in promoting growth and disease resistance

Vitamin B_{12} and Folic Acid

Act with vit. E in treatment of macrocytic anemia

Vit. E can substitute for or potentiate vit. B_{12}

Vitamin K and CoQ

Very similar in structure to vit. E

Pantothenic acid—Promotes synthesis of vit. E in plants

2. Relationship to Hormones

FSH and LH—Production increased in vit. E deficiency

Testosterone—Testicular degeneration due to vit. E deficiency in rats causes decreased production of testosterone

High content of vit. E in testicular tissues, seminal fluid

Cortisone—Requirements for cortisone and vit. E increase during stress. High content of vit. E at sites of cortisone synthesis in adrenal cortex

STH—A synergist in growth

3. Unusual Features

May be involved in aging mechanisms by protecting unsaturated fatty acids and membranes against free radicals

Only d-isomers occur naturally

Vitamin E replaceable by selenium salts in therapy of rat and pig liver necrosis, and chick exudative diathesis

Vitamin E replaceable by CoQ and antioxidants for certain symptoms of vit. E deficiency but not for all, e.g., RBC hemolysis, resorption gestation not affected.

Species differences in response to vit. E treatment of similar symptoms, e.g. muscular dystrophy—rabbits positive, humans negative

Other tocopherols only slightly active compared to vit. E

Decreased in tumors

4. Possible Relationships of Deficiency Symptoms to Metabolic Action

Muscular dystrophy, creatinuria (rabbit, monkey)—Maintenance of muscle cell membranes

RBC hemolysis (man)—Maintenance of red cell membranes

Fetal resorption (rats)—Maintenance of uterine membranes and uterine nerve ganglia

Mycardial degeneration (dog, rabbit)—Maintenance of muscle cell membranes

Steatorrhea (man)—Impaired lipid absorption by intestinal cells; maintenance of intestinal cell membranes

Encephalomalacia (chick)—Maintenance of nerve and membrane structures

6
Vitamin K

GENERAL INFORMATION

1. **Synonyms:** Antihemorrhagic vitamin, prothrombin factor, Koagulations-vitamin

2. **History**
   - 1929—Dam reported chicks on synthetic diet develop hemorrhagic conditions
   - 1935—Dam named vit. K as the missing factor in synthetic diet
   - 1935—Almquist and Stokstad demonstrated vit. K present in fish meal and alfalfa
   - 1939—Dam and Karrer isolated vit. K from alfalfa
   - 1939—Doisy isolated K_1 from alfalfa, K_2 from fish meal, and demonstrated difference
   - 1939—MacCorquodale, Cheney, Fieser determined structure of vit. K_1
   - 1939—Almquist and Klose synthesized vit. K_1
   - 1941—Link *et al.* discovered dicoumarol

3. **Physiological Forms**
   - Plant—Vitamin K_1 (phylloquinone, phytonadione)
   - Animal—Vitamin $K_{2(20)}$.
   - Bacterial—Vitamin K_2 (farnoquinone) ($K_{2(30)}$, $K_{2(35)}$)

4. **Active Analogs and Related Compounds**
   - Menadiol diphosphate, menadione (vit. K_3), menadione bisulfite
   - Phthiocol, synkayvite, menadiol (vit. K_4), vits. K_5, K_6, K_7

5. **Inactive Analogs and Related Compounds:**   Reduced vit. K

6. **Antagonists:**   Dicoumarol,   sulfonamides,   antibiotics, α-tocopherol quinone, dihydroxystearic acid glycide, salicylates, iodinin, warfarin

7. **Synergists:**   Vitamins E, A, C; STH

8. **Physiological Functions:**   Prothrombin synthesis in liver, blood-clotting mechanisms, electron transport mechanisms, growth, photosynthetic mechanisms

9. **Deficiency Diseases, Disorders:**   Hypoprothrombinemia

10. **Sources for Species Requiring It:**
    Many species require it
    Exogenous sources: Vertebrates, some bacteria. (Intestinal bacteria provide in man)
    Endogenous sources: Plants, bacteria, and all other organisms requiring it

CHEMISTRY

1. **Structure**

Vitamin K_1, $C_{31}H_{46}O_2$

2. **Reactions**

Heat—Stable	Oxidation—Stable
Acid—(Strong) labile	Reduction—Labile
Alkali—Labile	Light—Labile
Water—Insol.	

3. **Properties**

	Important Groups for activity
Appearance—Yellow oil	Menadiol nucleus
MW—450.7	Phytyl side chain
MP— −20°C	*Trans*-methyl groups
Crystal Form—No data	
Salts—Disodium phosphate	

Solubility

H$_2$O—Insol.

Acet., Alc.—Sol.

Benz. Chl. Eth.—Sol.

Absn. Max.—243, 249, 260,

269, 325 mμ (hexane)

Chemical Nature: Quinone

$\alpha_D^{20} = -0.4°C$ (benzene)

4. Commercial Production: Column Chromatography of fish meal extracts

5. Isolation

Sources—Fish meal, alfalfa

Method

Remove chlorophyll from pet. ether extract by column chromatography on ZnCO$_3$

Reduce to hydroquinone using sodium hydrosulfite

Extract with pet. ether, alkali, ether

Oxidize hydroquinone to quinone

6. Determination

Bioassay—Vitamin K deficient chick assay

Physicochemical—Polarographic methods; spectrophotometry of pure solutions; prothrombin time determination

DISTRIBUTION AND SOURCES

1. Occurrence

Plants:

Fruit—Orange (peel), tomato

Vegetables—Spinach, cabbage, brussel sprouts, alfalfa, cauliflower, soybean (oil)

Nuts and seeds—Hemp seed

Animals: Pork liver, eggs, milk, fish meal

Microorganisms: Intestinal bacteria, *M. phlei*

2. Dietary Sources

High: 100-300 μg/100 g

Cabbage, cauliflower, soybeans, spinach

Pork, Beef liver, beef kidney

Medium: 10-100 μg/100 g

Potatoes, strawberries, tomatoes, alfalfa, wheat (whole, germ, bran), pine needles, egg yolk

Low: 0-10 μg/100 g

Corn, carrots, peas, parsley, mushrooms, milk

MEDICAL AND NUTRITIONAL ROLE

1. **Units:**   0.0008 mg menadione = 20 dam units = 1 ansbacher unit

2. **Normal Blood Levels (Man):**   Not reported

3. **Recommended Allowances**
   Children—Supplied by intestinal bacteria normally
   Adults—Supplied by intestinal bacteria normally
   Special
       Increases with external temperature
       Newborn infants with neonatal hemorrhage
       Mothers in labor
       Overdosage with anticoagulants

4. **Administration**
   Injection—Intravenous, intramuscular
   Topical—No data
   Oral—Occasionally

5. **Factors Affecting Availability**
   Decrease
       Biliary obstruction
       Liver damage—cirrhosis, toxins
       Poor food preparation conditions
       Presence of antagonists
       Impaired lipid absorption in gut
       Ingestion of mineral oil
       Sterilization of gut with antibiotics and sulfa drugs
       Excretion in feces
   Increase
       Storage in liver
       Absorption aids—bile salts

6. **Deficiency Symptoms**
   Hypoprothrombinemia—General
   Increased bleeding and hemorrhage—General
   Increased clotting time—General
   Neonatal hemorrhage—General
   Internal hemorrhage (chick)

7. **Effects of Overdose**
   Usually nontoxic, occasionally toxic
   Possible thrombosis, vomiting, porphyrinuria—man
   Albuminuria—dog
   Increased clotting time—rabbit
   Cytopenia, hemoglobinemia—mouse
   Kernicterus (menadione)

METABOLIC ROLE

1. **Biosynthesis**
   Precursors—Polyacetic acid (ring); acetate (side chain)
   Intermediates—Dehydroquinic acid (ring); farnesol (side chain)

2. **Production:**   Species and sites
   Plants—green leaves
   Bacteria—intestinal (main source)

3. **Storage Sites:**   Liver (small)

4. **Blood Carriers:**   Lipoproteins

5. **Half-life:**   Depletion causes deficiency within 10 days in rat

6. **Target tissues:**   Liver, vascular system

7. **Reactions**
   Coenzyme form—Vitamin $K_{2(20)}$, CoQ(?)

Organ	Enzyme System	Effect
	Electron transport	
Bacteria	Malate reductase	Activated
Bacteria	DPNH dehydrogenase	Activated
Liver	Vit. K reductase	Reduction of vit. K
Liver	Oxidative phosphorylation	Completes system
Liver	Respiratory chain	Completes system

8. **Mode of Action**
     Cellular
          Anabolic
               Prothrombin synthesis (liver)
               β-Globulin synthesis (liver)
               Photosynthesis-Hill reaction
          Catabolic—Decreases phosphate incorporation into liver RNA
          Other—Mitochondrial electron transport systems component
     Organismal
          Maintenance of prothrombin and clotting factors VII, IX, X
          Control internal hemorrhage
          Anabolic—Increase nitrogen retention

9. **Catabolism**
     Intermediates—Lactones
     Excretion products—As glucuronide and sulfate conjugates in urine, bile, feces

MISCELLANEOUS

1. **Relationship to Other Vitamins**
     Vitamin E—Synergistic to vit. K—Maintains reduced state similar in structure to vit. K_1 and probably interconvertible by way of CoQ and ubichromenols
     Vitamins A and C—Fragility of RBC correlated with vits. A, C, K

2. **Relationship to Hormones**
     STH—Synergist in growth

3. **Unusual Features**
     Intestinal absorption of vit. K in chicks poor
     Side chains of vit. K identical to those in ubiquinones (CoQ)
     Completely supplied by intestinal flora in normal adults
     Vitamin K lost on γ-irradiation of foods

4. **Possible Relationships of Deficiency Symptoms to Metabolic Action**
     Hemorrhage—Decreased synthesis of prothrombin and other clotting factors by the liver

7
Thiamine

GENERAL INFORMATION

1. Synonyms: Vitamin B_1, aneurin, antineuritic factor, antiberiberi factor, oryzamin

2. History
- 1897—Eijkman ameliorated beriberi in humans by addition of rice polishings to diet
- 1911—Funk isolated dietary growth factor from rice polishings which cured beriberi; coined term "vitamine"
- 1915—McCollum and Davis proposed term "water-soluble B" for antiberiberi factor
- 1920—Emmet and Luros demonstrated two growth factors in rice polishings, including antiberiberi factor destroyed by autoclaving
- 1926—Jansen and Donath isolated crystalline antiberiberi factor from rice bran
- 1927—Brit. Med. Res. Council proposed name of B_1 for antiberiberi factor
- 1936—Williams synthesized B_1 and named it thiamine

3. Physiological Forms
- Thiamine pyrophosphate (cocarboxylase)—Animals
- Thiamine orthophosphate—Animals
- Free thiamine—Plants

4. **Active Analogs and Related Compounds**
   Ethyl substituted for methyl on pyrimidine C-2
   Thiamine disulfide, acylated thiamine

5. **Inactive Analogs and Related Compounds:**   Reduced thiamine

6. **Antagonists:**   Pyrithiamine, oxythiamine, 2-n-butyl homologue

7. **Synergists:**   Vitamins B_{12}, B_2, B_6, niacin, pantothenic acid, STH

8. **Physiological Functions:**   Coenzyme in pyruvate metabolism; growth,
   appetite, digestion, nerve activity, gastrointestinal tonus, carbohydrate metabolism, energy production

9. **Deficiency Diseases, Disorders:**   Beriberi, opisthotonos (in birds), polyneuritis, hyperesthesia, bradycardia, edema

10. **Sources for Species Requiring It**
    All species require it for life
    Exogenous sources—All animals, some (algae, fungi, bacteria). Not much
        available from intestinal bacteria in man, although it is made there
    Endogenous sources—Some (algae, fungi, bacteria), all higher plants.
        Sheep and cattle get sufficiency from intestinal bacteria

CHEMISTRY

1. **Structure**

Thiamine hydrochloride,
$C_{12}H_{17}N_4OSCl \cdot HCl$

Pyrimidine   Thiazole

2. **Reactions**

Heat—Labile	Oxidation—Forms thiochrome
Acid—Stable	(fluoresc.)
Alkali—Unstable	Reduction—Unstable
Water—Acid (HCl)	Light—UV decomposes

3. **Properties**

Appearance—White
    crystals

MW—337.3 (as HCl)

MP—244°C

Crystal Form—
    Monocl. plates

Salts—Mononitrate,
    noble metals

Important Groups for activity
    —OH of —$CH_2 CH_2 OH$
    C-2 of pyrimidine
    C-2 of thiazole

Solubility
    H_2O—1 g/ml H_2O
    Alc.—sol.
    Acet. Benz., Chl., Eth.—Insol
    Absn. Max.—235, 267 mμ
    Chemical Nature—Base, alc.,
        substituted pyrimidine
    Misc.—Charact. odor
        pKa = 4.8, 9.2
    α_D = 0 (inactive)

4. **Commercial Production:**   Synthesis
Pyrimidine + thiazole nuclei synthesized separately and then condensed
Build on pyrimidine with acetamidine

5. **Isolation**
Sources—Rice bran, wheat germ, yeast
Method—Aqueous extraction, adsorption on Fuller's earth; elute with
quinine sulfate, precipitate as phosphotungstate, decompose precipitate and reprecipitate with $AuCl_3$, extract with water, precipitate from EtOH as hydrochloride

6. **Determination**
Bioassay—Yeast fermentation; polyneuritic rat—rate of cure; bacterial
metabolism
Physicochemical—Thiochrome fluorescence; polarographic; chroma-
tographic; absorption at 235-267 mμ in neutral solution; at 247 in
acid solution

DISTRIBUTION AND SOURCES

1. **Occurrence**
Plants
    Fruit—All. Low (except gooseberries, plums, which are medium)
    Vegetables—All. Low (except beans, green leafy types, cauliflower,
    corn, peas, potatoes—medium)
    Nuts—All. Medium (except coconut, which is low)
    Grains—All. Medium (except outer grain kernels, bran, polishings,
    wheat germ, which are high)

Animals: All—Medium (except pork, which is high, and some fish, which
    are low)
Microorganisms: Yeast (killed)—high. Intestinal bacteria not available
Misc.—Mushrooms—medium

2. Dietary Sources

High: 1000-10,000 μg/100 g
    Wheat germ, rice bran, soybean flour
    Yeast
    Ham
Medium: 100-1000 μg/100 g
    Gooseberries, plums, prunes (dry), raisins (dry), asparagus, beans
        (kidney, lima, snap, soy, wax), beet greens, broccoli, brussel
        sprouts, cauliflower, chicory, endive, corn, dandelion greens, kale,
        kohlrabi, leeks, lentils (dry), parsley, peas, potatoes, watercress,
        barley, oats, rice (brown), almonds, brazil, cashews, chestnuts,
        hazelnuts, peanuts, pecans, walnuts
    Beef, calf, chicken, pork, lamb, turkey meat and organs, mushrooms
    Eggs, milk, carp, clams, cod, lobster, mackerel, oysters, salmon
Low: 10-100 μg/100 g
    Apples, apricots, avocados, bananas, berries (black-, blue-, cran-, rasp-,
        straw-), melons (cantaloupe, water, honeydew), cherries, currants,
        dates (dry), figs, grapes, grapefruit, lemons, oranges, peaches, pears,
        pineapples, prunes, tangerines
    Artichokes, beets, cabbage, carrots, celery, cucumbers, eggplant,
        lettuce, onions, parsnips, peppers, pumpkins, radishes, rhubarb,
        spinach, sweet potatoes, turnips, coconut, cheeses, flounder
    Haddock, halibut, herring, pike, sardines, scallops, shrimp, trout, tuna

MEDICAL AND NUTRITIONAL ROLE

1. **Units:** 1 USP unit = 3 μg thiamine HCl = 1 I.U.

2. **Normal Blood Levels (Man):** 1.3 μg/100 free base in serum. 3-11 μg/100
    cocarboxylase in blood cells

3. **Recommended Allowances**
    Children—0.6-1.1 mg/day
    Adults—1.0 mg/day, female; 1.4 mg/day, male
    Special—Increased requirements in pregnancy and lactation. Depends on
        body weight, calorie intake, intestinal synthesis and absorption, fat
        content of diet (increased pyruvate)

4. **Administration**
    Injection—Intravenous, intraperitoneal
    Topical—No data
    Oral—Preferred route

5. **Factors Affecting Availability**
    Decrease
        Cooking—heat labile, water soluble
        Enzymes in food; thiaminase for vitamin breakdown
        Destruction by $CaCO_3$, K_2HPO_4, $MnSO_4$
        Nitrites, sulfites destroy
        Diuresis, gastrointestinal diseases
        Live yeast, alkali
    Increase
        Cellulose in diet increases intestinal synthesis
        Small storage capacity in heart, liver, kidney
        Bacterial synthesis in intestine (normally none)

6. **Deficiency Symptoms**
    General (Man); beriberi
        Anesthesia, hyperesthesia
        Retarded growth, neuron degeneration
        Fatigue, weight loss, anorexia, G.I. complaints, weakness, loss of
            reflexes, and vibratory sense
        Circulatory and cardiac involvement
        Mental disturbances—depression, irritability, memory loss
        Muscular atrophy in extremities
        Increased blood pyruvate and lactate
    Lab animals
        Decreased fat stores, decreased body temperature
        Neurological disturbance—polyneuritis, decrease in tone
        Bradycardia, cardiac enlargement, edema
        Opisthotonos (chickens, pigeons, turkey)

7. **Effects of Overdose**
    Humans—Limited toxicity, starting at approx. 125-350 mg/kg dosage.
        Edema, nervousness, sweating, tachycardia, tremors, herpes, allerg-
        icity, fatty liver, vascular hypotension
    Rats—Sterility, B_6 Deficiency

METABOLIC ROLE

1. **Biosynthesis**
   Precursors—Thiazole, pyrimidine pyrophosphate
   Intermediates—Thiamine phosphate

2. **Production Sites**
   Plants—Grain and cereal germ
   Bacteria—Intestinal

3. **Storage Sites:** Heart, liver, kidney, brain (all small amounts)

4. **Blood Carriers:** Blood cells—As cocarboxylase. Serum—free B_1

5. **Half-life:** 1 mg/day destroyed in tissues

6. **Target Tissues:** Heart, liver, kidney, peripheral nerves, brain

7. **Reactions**
   Coenzyme Forms—cocarboxylase (thiamine pyrophosphate, disphospho-thiamine). Needs Mg^{++} ion

Organ	Enzyme System	Effect
Liver, plants	Transketolase	Activated
Serum	Choline esterase	Inhibited
Liver, yeast	Thiaminokinase—thiamine → cocarboxylase	Activated
Plants	Decarboxylases: Nonoxidate decarboxylation of pyruvate to OAA	Activated
Liver (mammals)	Oxidative decarboxylation of pyruvate with lipoic acid	Activated
Liver (mammals)	Phosphoroclastic cleavage of α-keto acids	Activated
Liver (mammals)	Formation of acetoin	Activated
Liver (mammals)	Oxidative decarboxylation of α-ketoglutarate to succinate	Activated

8. **Mode of Action**
   Cellular
   Anabolic—Condensations, synthesis of acetylcholine
   Catabolic—α-Keto acid decarboxylation (Krebs cycle coenzyme—ATP generation), oxidations, dismutations
   Other—Transketolation, formation of NADPH, and ribose via HMP shunt, acyl transfer agent—"active" acetaldehyde

Organismal
   Maintenance of nerve tissues
   Maintenance of heart muscle
   Decrease blood pyruvate and lactate
   Maintain supply of ATP
   Normal growth maintenance

9. **Catabolism:** Intermediates—Pyrimidine. Excretion products—Pyrimidine and thiamine

MISCELLANEOUS

1. **Relationship to Other Vitamins**
   Vitamin B_{12} —Synergistic to B_1
   Pantothenic Acid, Niacin, Riboflavin—Energy from oxidation of carbohydrates depends on synergism with thiamine (oxidative decarboxylation)
   Vitamin C—Decreases requirement for B_1
   Vitamin B_6 —Overdose of B_1 causes B_6 deficiency in rats
   Vitamin D—Tolerance increased by vit. B_1
   Riboflavin, Pyridoxine—Synergize with thiamine to produce niacin

2. **Relationship to Hormones**
   Acetylcholine—Synthesis requires vit. B_1
   Thyroxine—Metabolic rate increase in hyperthyroidism increases B_1 requirement
   Insulin—In diabetes B_1 content of blood and liver reduced
   STH—Synergist in growth

3. **Unusual features**
   Hormonal function in plants—controls root growth
   Phosphorylation in liver, dephosphorylation in kidney
   Vitamin B enzymes easily poisoned by heavy metals, mustard gas, acetyl iodide
   Plant and animal cocarboxylases identical
   Has a diuretic effect, is constipative
   Can be allergenic on injection
   Blood contains most cocarboxylase in leukocytes
   Thiamine sparing action by alcohol, fat, protein
   Not available from intestinal bacteria

4. Possible Relationships of Deficiency to Metabolic Action

Flooding of system with pyruvate
   Weight loss
   G.I. complaints
   Fatigue
   Anorexia
Decreased synthesis of acetylcholine
   Polyneuritis
   Mental disturbances
   Circulatory and cardiac involvement

8
Riboflavin

GENERAL INFORMATION

1. Synonyms: Vitamin B_2, vit. G, lactoflavin, hepatoflavin, ovoflavin, verdo-flavin, 6,7-dimethyl-9-(d-1'-ribityl)isoalloxazine

2. History

1917—Emmet and McKim showed dietary growth factor for rats in rice polishings

1920—Emmett suggested presence of several dietary growth factors in yeast concentrate, including heat-stable component and B_1

1927—Brit. Med. Res. Council proposed name of B_2 for heat-stable component

1932—Warburg and Christian isolated yellow enzyme (containing riboflavin (FMN)) from bottom yeast

1933—Kuhn isolated pure B_2 (riboflavin) from milk; recognized growth promoting activity

1935—Kuhn *et al.*; Karrer *et al.*—Achieved structure and synthesis of vit. B_2; named it riboflavin

1954—Christie *et al.* determined structure and synthesized FAD

3. Physiological Forms: Riboflavin mononucleotide (FMN). Riboflavin dinucleotide (FAD)

4. Active Analogs and Related Compounds: 7-Methyl-9-methyl, and 6-ethyl-7-methyl compounds, arabinoflavin

5. **Inactive   Analogs   and   Related   Compounds:**   3,6,7-Trimethyl-9-(d-1'-ribityl)isoalloxazine

6. **Antagonists:** Isoriboflavin, lumiflavin, araboflavin, hydroxyethyl analogue, formyl methyl analogue, galactoflavin, flavin mono-SO_4

7. **Synergists:** Vitamins A, B_1, B_6, B_{12}, niacin, pantothenic acid, folic acid, biotin, T4, insulin, STH

8. **Physiological Functions**
   Coenzyme in respiratory enzyme systems
   Constituent of flavoproteins, redox systems, respiratory enzymes
   Growth and development of fetus
   Maintenance of mucosal, epithelial, and eye tissues

9. **Deficiency Diseases, Disorders:** Glossitis, cheilosis, seborrheic dermatitis, corneal vascularization, anemia

10. **Sources for Species Requiring It**
    All organisms require it
    Endogenous sources—Higher plants, algae, some bacteria, some fungi
    Exogenous sources—All animals, some fungi and bacteria (intestinal bacteria make it, but most is unavailable to man)

CHEMISTRY

1. **Structure**

Riboflavin, $C_{17}H_{20}O_6N_4$

Purine

2. **Reactions**

Heat—Blackens at 240°C
Acid—Stable
Alkali—Labile → lumiflavin
Water—Soluble, acidic

Oxidation—Decomposes
Reduction—Easily → leucoribo-
  flavin
Light—Photolyses to lumiflavin
  Intense green fluorescence
  565 mμ

3. **Properties**

Appearance—Orange-yellow
  powder
MW—376.4
MP—282°C
Crystal Form—Needles
Salts—Borate, PO_4, acetate

Important Groups
  9-N, 5'-OH
  6,7-methyl
  3-N

Solubility
  H_2O—Sol. 0.01 g/100 ml
  Acet., Alc.—Insol.
  Benz., Chl., Eth.—Insol.
  Absn. Max.—220, 267, 336,
    446 mμ
Misc.—pI = 6
  $[\alpha]_D^{20}$ = −114° (0.1 N NaOH)
Chemical Nature
  Reducing agent; nucleotide
  Substituted purine

4. **Commercial Production**

Fermentation bacteria or yeast
Chemical synthesis from alloxan, ribose, and o-xylene

5. **Isolation**

Sources—Free—urine, whey, retina. Combined—as FMN or FAD—tissues
  or egg whites
Method
  Aq. extract of tissue treated with ether
  Fractional pptn. with picric acid
  Ppt. out proteins with ammon sulfate
  Adsorb on Fuller's earth
  Elute with 0.1 N NaOH
  Crystallize from aq. pet. ether-acetone mixture

6. **Determination**

Bioassay—Rats—growth rate. Microbiological—*L caseii, L. mesenteroides*
Physicochemical—Fluorimetry, paper electrophoresis, polarography

DISTRIBUTION AND SOURCES

1. **Occurrence**
    Plants
        Fruit—All. Low
        Vegetables—All. High in tomato leaves. Medium in green leafy types,
        corn, cauliflower, beans. Low in others
        Nuts—All. Medium except coconut (low)
        Flowers—Saffron (high)
    Animals—All (liver > kidneys > heart > other tissues). High in organs,
        medium in other tissues. Crustaceans—High
    Microorganisms: All, esp. yeast, anerobic bacteria (high)

2. **Dietary Sources**
    High: 1000-10,000 μg/100 g
        Beef (kidneys, liver), calf (kidney, liver)
        Chicken (liver)
        Pork (heart, kidneys, liver), sheep (liver, kidneys)
        Yeast (killed)
    Medium: 100-1000 μg/100 g
        Avocados, currants
        Asparagus, beans (kidney, lima, snap, wax), beet greens, broccoli,
        brussel sprouts, cauliflower, chicory, endive, corn, dandelion greens,
        kale, kohlrabi, lentils (dry), parsley, parsnips, peas, soybeans (dry),
        spinach, turnip greens, watercress, almonds (dry), cashews, peanuts,
        pecans, walnuts, rice bran, wheat germ, oats, cheeses, cream, eggs,
        milk
        Bacon, beef, chicken, duck, goose, pork, lamb, turkey, veal, fish
    Low: 10-100 μg/100 g
        Apples, apricots, bananas, blackberries, blueberries, cranberries, rasp-
        berries, strawberries, cherries, grapes, grapefruit, melons, oranges,
        peaches, dates (dry), figs, pears, pineapples, plums, raisins (dry),
        tangerines, artichokes, beets, cabbages, carrots, celery, cucumbers,
        eggplant, lettuce, onions, peppers, potatoes, pumpkins, radishes,
        sweet potatoes, tomatoes, turnips, coconuts, barley, rice

MEDICAL AND NUTRITIONAL ROLE

1. **Units:** By weight, μg or mg

2. **Normal Blood Levels:** 6.6 μg/100 ml

3. **Recommended Allowances**
    Children—0.6-1.2 mg/day*
    Adults—1.5 mg/day female*; 1.7 mg/day male*

4. **Administration**
    Injection—I.V.
    Topical—No data
    Oral—Preferred route

5. **Factors Affecting Availability**
    Decrease
        Cooking (sl. sol. in H_2O)
        Plant foods—Lower availability, bound forms
        Decreased phosphorylation in intestines prevents absorption
        Exposure of foods to sunlight
        Enzymes for breakdown
        Gastrointestinal disease
        Diuresis
    Increase
        Storage in heart, liver and kidneys
        Very actively producing intestinal bacteria (small amount)

6. **Deficiency Symptoms**
    General
        Orogenital syndrome
        Stomatitis
        Glossitis
        Cheilosis
        Seborrheic dermatitis
        Ocular—Photophobia, indistinct vision, corneal vascularity increased
    Rats
        Poor growth, ocular abnormality
        Dermatitis (eczema—nostrils, eyes)
        Myelin degeneration, testicular atrophy
        Thymus involution
    Dogs
        Weight loss, fatty liver, muscle weakness
        Opacity of corneal epithelium

---

* Related to caloric intake and protein levels. Increased in pregnancy, lactation. Additional sources in intestinal bacteria (small).

Chicken
Egg production and hatchability decline, nerve degeneration
Monkey
Anemia, leukopenia

7. **Effects of Overdose**
Essentially nontoxic in man
Anuria—rat
Azotemia—rat
Kidney insufficiency—rat
Paresthesia—man
Itching—man

METABOLIC ROLE

1. **Biosynthesis**
Precursors—Purines, pyrimidines, ribose
Intermediates—6,7-Dimethyl-8-ribityllumazine

2. **Production Site**
Plants—Leaves, germinating seeds, root nodules
Bacteria—Intestinal

3. **Storage Sites:** Heart, liver, kidneys (small amount)

4. **Blood carriers:** As nucleotides

5. **Half-life:** 12% of intake excreted in 24 hr

6. **Target Tissues:** Heart, liver, kidneys, others in lesser amount

7. **Reactions**
Coenzyme forms
Redox couple: oxidized ⇌ reduced form
FMN, FAD (binding to apoenzyme via cations (Fe^{++}, Cu^{++}, Mo^{++}) to PO_4 of coenzyme)

Organ	Enzyme System	Effect
Liver	(1) FMN—Warburg yellow enzyme, cytochrome C reductase, l-amino acid, oxidase succinic dehydrogenase	Activated
Liver	(2) FAD—Xanthine oxidase, d-amino acid oxidase, glycine oxidase, diaphorase, fumaric dehydrogenase, glucose oxidases, histaminases, aldehyde oxidase	Activated
Intestine	(3) Flavokinase—Phosphorylation of riboflavin	Activated

8. **Mode of Action**
   Cellular
     Anabolic—No data
     Catabolic—Carbohydrate metabolism
     Other—Essential complexed part of flavoproteins
       Mitochondrial electron transport system
       Oxidation-reduction enzyme systems
       Accepts 2H on isoalloxazine ring
       Part of respiratory enzyme system
   Organismal
     Ectodermal maintenance—skin and cornea
     Growth and development of fetus
     Maintenance of nervous system (myelin sheath)
     Resistance to disease

9. **Catabolism**
     Intermediates—No data
     Excretion products
       Urine—Free vitamin—Diurnal variations. Normally ~1/3 of dietary amounts excreted
       Feces—Uroflavin—Diurnal variations

MISCELLANEOUS

1. **Relationship to Other Vitamins**
     Vitamin A, Niacin—Present with riboflavin in visual structures (retina) involved in visual process
     Niacin—Riboflavin enzymes utilize DPN, and DPNH
     Thiamine—Deficiency of B_1 leads to increased storage of riboflavin. Involved with riboflavin in thyroxine and insulin utilization in CHO metabolism
     Other B vitamins—Synergistic with riboflavin

2. **Relationship to Hormones**

   ACTH—Riboflavin involved in release of ACTH from pituitary

   Thyroxine, Insulin—Effective only if riboflavin and thiamine are present

   Thyroxine—Incorporation of iodide by sheep thyroid stimulated by FMN

   Adrenal hormones—Aid in phosphorylation of riboflavin in intestines

   Estradiol—Inactivation in liver decreased in riboflavin deficiency (rat)

   STH—Synergist in growth

3. **Unusual Features**

   High levels in liver inhibit tumor formation by azo compounds in animals

   Free radicals formed by light or dehydrogenation: flavine ⇌ semi-quinone ⇌ dihydroflavin

   Free vitamin only in retina, urine, milk and semen

   Substitution of adenine by other purines, pyrimidines destroys activity of FAD

   Phosphorylation of vitamin in intestines allows absorption as FMN

   Blood levels decrease during life in humans

   Brain content remains constant

   Available in plants as FMN and FAD

   Concentrated in bull semen

4. **Possible Relationships of Deficiency Symptoms to Metabolic Action**

   Ectodermal manifestations related to other B-vitamin deficiencies

       Cheilosis

       Glossitis

       Stomatitis

       Seborrheic dermatitis

       Corneal vascularity

       Orogenital syndrome

   Synergistic functions of vit. A and riboflavin in visual structures—Photophobia

9
Vitamin B₆

GENERAL INFORMATION

1. **Synonyms:** Pyridoxine, adermine, pyridoxol

2. **History**

   1934—György cured a dermatitis in rats not due to B_1 or B_2 with yeast extract factor

   1938—Lepkovsky isolated similar factor from rice bran extract

   1938—Keresztesy and Stevens isolated and crystallized pure B_6 from rice polishings

   1938—Kohn, Wendt, and Westphal synthesized pyridoxine, gave pyridoxine its name

   1939—Stiller, Keresztesy, and Stevens established structure of pyridoxine

   1945—Snell discovered pyridoxal and pyridoxamine

   1953—Snyderman *et al*. first recognized and established B_6 requirement in humans

3. **Physiological Forms**

   Interconvertible *in vivo* (pyridoxine ⇌ pyridoxal ⇌ pyridoxamine)

   Animals—Pyridoxal-5-phosphate (codecarboxylase); pyridoxamine phosphate

   Plants—Pyridoxol-5-phosphate, pyridoxal-5-P, pyridoxamine-P

4. **Active Analogs and Related Compounds:** Pyridoxal, pyridoxamine

5. **Inactive Analogs and Related Compounds:** Nor-vitamin B$_6$, 4-pyridoxic acid, 5-pyridoxic acid

6. **Antagonists:** 4-deoxypyridoxine, 4-methoxypyridoxine, toxopyrimidine, penicillamine, semicarbazide, isoniazid

7. **Synergists:** Vitamins B$_1$, B$_2$, C, E, niacin, biotin, folic acid, STH, glucagon, epinephrine, norepinephrine

8. **Physiological Functions**
   Protein, CHO, and lipid metabolism
   Coenzyme in many phases of amino acid metabolism; especially in gluconeogenesis, production of neural hormones, bile acids, unsaturated fatty acids, and porphyrins
   Erythrocyte formation, growth

9. **Deficiency Diseases, Disorders**
   Monkey—Arteriosclerosis
   Rats—Acrodynia
   Man—Lymphopenia, convulsions, dermatitis, irritability, nervous disorders

10. **Sources for Species Requiring It**
    All animals require B$_6$
    Exogenous sources—Animals, some bacteria (intestinal bacteria make it, but not much is available to man)
    Endogenous sources—Plants, fungi, intestinal bacteria

CHEMISTRY

1. **Structures**

Pyridoxine, C$_8$H$_{11}$NO$_3$ Pyridoxal   Pyridoxamine

2. Reactions

Heat—Stable
Acid—Stable
Alkali—Stable
Water—Basic

Oxidation—Unstable
Reduction—Unstable
Light—Labile (stable in acid)

3. Properties

Appearance—White powder
MW—169 pyridoxine
MP—160° pyridoxine
Crystal Form—Platelets
Salts—Hydrochloride, Ca^{++}
Important Groups for activity
    $-CH_2OH$
    $-N=$

Solubility
  H_2O—0.2 g/ml
  Acet., Alc.—Sol.
  Benz., Chl., Eth.—Insol.
  Absn. Max.—256, 327 mμ
  pH 7.0
Chemical Nature
  hydroxylated weak nitrogen base,
  substituted pyridine
pKa = 5.0, 8.9
αD = 0 (inactive)

4. Commercial Production

Commercially available as pyridoxine hydrochloride
Synthesized by method of Harris and Folkers. Ethoxy acetylacetone
    condensed with cyanoacetamide
Easiest route for synthesis is probably from oxazoles

5. Isolation

Sources—Rice polishings or bran and yeast
Methods
    Adsorption on Fuller's earth or charcoal
    Elute with $Ba(OH)_2$
    Precipitate impurities with heavy metals
    Precipitation with phosphotungstic acid

6. Determination

Bioassay—Animal
    Rat acrodynia test
    Rat growth and chicken growth assays
    Tryptophane loading test
    Blood cell
Bioassay—Microbial—Microbioassay
Physicochemical—Photofluorometric procedure detects 4-pyridoxic acid-
    (major metabolite) in urine. Chromatographic procedure to detect
    4-pyridoxic acid

DISTRIBUTION AND SOURCES

1. **Occurrence**
   Plants
      Fruit—All low, except bananas, avocados, grapes, pears (medium)
      Vegetables—All low or medium
      Nuts—All high
      Misc.—Cereals—medium, except brown rice, wheat germ (high); and
         blackstrap molasses (high)
   Animals: All medium, except herring, salmon, liver (high)
   Microorganisms: All high or medium—yeast, intestinal bacteria (high);
         some other bacteria

2. **Dietary Sources**
   High: 1000-10,000 µg/100 g
      Liver (beef, calf, pork), herring, salmon
      Walnuts, peanuts, wheat germ, brown rice
      Yeast, blackstrap molasses
   Medium: 100-1000 µg/100 g
      Bananas, avocados, grapes, pears
      Barley, cabbage, carrots, corn, oats, peas, potatoes, rye, kale,
         tomatoes, turnips, yams, brussel sprouts, cauliflower, spinach,
         soybeans, wheat
      Beef, lamb, pork, veal (heart, brains, kidney); cod, flounder, halibut,
         mackerel, whale, sardines, tuna
      Butter, eggs
   Low: 10-100 µg/100 g
      Apples, cantaloupes, grapefruit, lemons, oranges, peaches, raisins,
         strawberries, watermelons, cherries, currants (red)
      Asparagus, beans, beet greens, lettuce, onions
      Cheese, milk

MEDICAL AND NUTRITIONAL ROLE

1. **Units:**   By weight, mg

2. **Normal Blood Levels:**   11.2 ug/100 ml

3. **Recommended Allowances**
      Children—0.5-1.2 mg/day*
      Adults—2.0 mg/day*
      Special—Pregnancy and lactation, 2.5 mg/day

* Depends on protein content of food and inborn errors of metabolism; irradiation increases
need.

4. **Administration**
    Injection—Intravenous, subcutaneous
    Topical—No data
    Oral—Preferred route

5. **Factors Affecting Availability**
    Decrease
        Administration of isoniazid
        30-45% loss in cooking, water sol.
        Diuresis, G.I. diseases
        Irradiation
    Increase
        Intestinal bacterial production (very small amount)
        Storage in liver

6. **Deficiency Symptoms**
    General
        Cutaneous lesions
        Anemia
        Neuronal dysfunction including convulsions
        Increased excretion of xanthurenic acid
    Lab Animals
        Blood urea and urea excretion enhanced
        γ-globulin and hemoglobin decreased
        Urinary oxalate increased
        Insulin insufficiency
        Acrodynia
        Demyelinization of peripheral nerves
        Tonoclonic convulsion
        Adrenal—enlarged zona fasciculata
        Poor reproduction

7. **Effects of Overdose**
    Limited toxicity man (only at 3 g/kg dosage)
    Convulsions at 4 g/kg (rat)

METABOLIC ROLE

1. **Biosynthesis**
    Precursors—Possibly glycine, serine or glycolaldehyde
    Intermediates—Unknown

2. **Production:** Species and Site
   Plants—Fungi, cereal germ, seeds
   Bacteria—Intestinal
   Animals—None

3. **Storage Site:** Muscle phosphorylase (skeletal muscle) (small amount)

4. **Blood Carriers:** Blood protein complexes

5. **Half-life:** 57% of ingested dose excreted per day

6. **Target Tissues:** Nervous tissue, liver, lymph nodes, muscle tissue

7. **Reactions**
   Coenzyme forms—Codecarboxylase (pyridoxal-5-phosphate); pyridoxamine phosphate; Cu, Fe, Al chelates of coenzymes probably are
   active forms

Organ	Enzyme System	Effect
Liver	1. Transaminases (glutamic, aspartic)	Activated
Liver	2. Amino acid decarboxylases (histidine)	Activated
Liver	3. Tryptophan metabolism (kynureninase)	Activated
Liver	4. Tyrosine and phenylalanine metabolism	Activated
Muscle	5. Phosphorylases (constituent of)	Completed
Liver	6. Dehydrases (porphyrin synthesis, serine)	Activated
Liver	7. Racemases (alanine racemase)	Activated
Liver	8. Oxidases (diamine)	Activated
Liver	9. Desulfhydrases (cysteine)	Activated
Liver	10. Serine transhydroxymethylase	Activated

8. **Mode of Action**
   Cellular
   Anabolic—Unsaturated fatty acid biosynthesis
   Catabolic—Nonoxidative metabolic changes, decarboxylations, trans-
   aminations, glycogen phosphorylation
   Other—amino acid absorption and transport
   Organismal
   Growth, maintenance of adrenal cortex
   Production of niacin, norepinephrine, serotonin, histamine, acetyl-
   choline, γ-aminobutyric acid

Production of bile acids (taurine synthesis)

Erythrocyte formation, gluconeogenesis and glycogenolysis reactions

9. Catabolism

Intermediates—All converted to pyridoxal

Excretion products

Urine—4-pyridoxic acid (3-4 mg/day); pyridoxal (0.2-0.3 mg/day)

Feces—0.5-0.8 mg/day

MISCELLANEOUS

1. Relationship to Other Vitamins

Pantothenic acid—B_6 defic. results in lowered concentration of coenzyme A

B_{12}—B_6 defic. results in reduced absorption and storage of B_{12}

Vitamin E—B_6 synergizes with E to control metabolism of unsaturated fats

Vitamin C—Excretion of C increased in B_6 deficiency, conversion of vit. C to oxalates increased, i.e., oxaluria. Helps alleviate some symptoms of B_6 deficiency. Synergizes with B_6 in tyrosine metabolism

Niacin—B_6 coenzyme for niacin synthesis from tryptophan, also synergistic

Vitamin B_1—Overdose of B_1 causes B_6 deficiency in rats, synergistic

Vitamin B_2—Synergistic in action with B_6

Biotin—Synergistic with B_6, B_2 and niacin in skin maintenance

2. Relationship to Hormones

Thyroxine—decreases the activity of various pyridoxalphosphate dependent enzyme systems

Insulin—Insufficiency of insulin in B_6 deficiency in animals

Norepinephrine, Acetylcholine, serotonin, epinephrine—B_6 involved in synthesis of these hormones

ACTH—Adrenal cortex zona fasciculata enlarged (hypertrophied) on B_6 deficiency

B_6 possibly involved in synthesis and function of these hormones (STH a synergist in growth)

STH

Estradiol-17β

Testosterone

FSH

LH

Cortisol
Aldosterone
Epinephrine
Glucagon

3. Unusual Features

Involved in dental caries, oxaluria

Linoleic acid relieves dermatitis symptoms of B$_6$ deficiency

Presence of B$_6$ in phosphorylase a and b in large amounts implicates glucagon, epinephrine, and norepinephrine in function of B$_6$

Great diversity of deficiency symptoms depending on species

Heavy metal ion involved in binding to enzyme

Involvement in stress, electrolyte balance, energy production, and water metabolism by unknown pathways

4. Possible Relationships of Deficiency Symptoms to Metabolic Action

Cutaneous lesions—Synergism of B$_6$ with niacin and B$_2$ for skin maintenance

Convulsions—Synergism of B$_6$ with B$_1$ involved in nervous tissue maintenance

Xanthurenic acid excretion—Kynureninase requires B$_6$ as coenzyme

Anemia—Synergism of B$_6$ with B$_{12}$ for anti-anemic action, maintenance of erythrocyte production

GENERAL INFORMATION

1. **Synonyms:** Cobalamin, cyanocobalamin

2. **History**
    1926—Minot and Murphy controlled pernicious anemia using liver
    1944—Castle demonstrated intrinsic factor needed to control pernicious anemia with liver
    1948—Rickes *et al.* isolated and crystallized factor in liver controlling pernicious anemia
    1948—Smith and Parker crystallized and designated liver factor as vit. B$_{12}$
    1948—West demonstrated clinical activity of vit. B$_{12}$
    1955—Hodgkin *et al.* determined structure of vit. B$_{12}$

3. **Physiological Forms:** Hydroxocobalamin (vit. B$_{12a}$). Aquocobalamin (vit. B$_{12b}$)

4. **Active Analogs and Related Compounds**
    Nitrocobalamin (vit. B$_{12c}$), chlorocobalamin, thiocyanatocobalamin

5. **Inactive Analogs and Related Compounds (in Man)**
    ψ-Vitamin B, factors B, C, D, E, F, G, H, I

6. **Antagonists:** Methylamide, ethylamide, anilide, lactone derivatives, pteridine, nicotinamide

7. **Synergists:**   Vitamins A, E, C, B$_1$, folic acid, biotin, pantothenic acid,

8. **Physiological Functions**
    Coenzyme in nucleic acid, protein and lipid synthesis
    Maintain growth, nucleic acid synthesis, protein synthesis, lipid synthesis, and methylations
    Maintain epithelial cells and nervous system (myelin sheath), erythropoiesis (with folic acid) and leukopoiesis

9. **Deficiency Diseases, Disorders:**   Retarded growth, pernicious anemia, megaloblastic anemia, macrocytic, hyperchromic anemia, glossitis, spinal cord degeneration, sprue

10. **Sources for Species Requiring It**
    Required by most vertebrates, some protozoa, bacteria, algae
    Exogenous sources—Vertebrates, some bacteria, protozoa, algae (not available from intestinal bacteria in man)
    Endogenous sources—Bacteria, actinomycetes

CHEMISTRY

1. **Structure**

Vitamin B$_{12}$,
$C_{63}H_{90}CoN_{14}O_{14}P$

2. Reactions

Heat—Unstable   Oxidation—Unstable
Acid—Unstable   Reduction—Unstable
Alkali—Unstable   Light—Unstable
Water—Neutral

3. Properties

Appearance—red powder   Solubility
MW—1357 H_2O—1.25 g/100 ml
MP—Blackens at $190°C$ Alc.—sol.
Crystal Form—Orthorhombic   Acet., Benz., Chl., Eth.—Insol.
  needles   Absn. Max.—278, 361,
Salts—Perchloric acid   550 mμ (H_2O)
Important Groups for activity $[\alpha]_D^{23}$ = $-59°$ (aq. soln.)
  5,6-Dimethylbenzimidazole   Chemical Nature
  α-Ribothiazole   Polyacidic base
                                      Benzimidazole nucleotide
                                      Porphyrin-like corrin
                                      Reducing agent

4. Commercial Production

Fermentation of *S. griseus* or *S. aureofaciens*
By-product of antibiotic production

5. Isolation

Sources—Liver, fish solubles
Method
  Extract with aqueous alcohol
  Adsorb B_{12} on charcoal, elute with 65% alcohol
  Column chromatography on silica or alumina
  Wash with acetone, elute with alcohol
  Crystallize

6. Determination

Bioassay
  Microbial—*L. leichmanii, O. malhamensis, E. gracilis*
  Animal—Chick and rat—curative dose
Physicochemical—Spectrophotometry, polarography, isotope dilution

DISTRIBUTION AND SOURCES

1. **Occurrence**

   Plants: Vegetables—Very low—soybeans, green beans, beets, carrots, peas
   Nuts, seeds—Very low—oats, wheat

   Animals: All animals, especially in organs—Liver, kidney, heart, spleen, brain, stomach, intestine
   Eggs, milk

   Microorganisms: *S. aureofaciens, B. megatherium,* protozoa, soil bacteria, intestinal bacteria

   Miscellaneous: Sea water, sewage sludge

2. **Dietary Sources**

   High: 50 μg-500 μg/100 g
   Kidney (lamb, beef)
   Liver (lamb, beef, calf, pork)
   Brain (beef)

   Medium: 5-50 μg/100 g
   Kidney (rabbit)
   Liver (rabbit, chicken)
   Heart (beef, rabbit, chicken)
   Egg yolk
   Clams, sardines, salmon, crabs, oysters, herring

   Low: 0.5-5 μg/100 g
   Cod, flounder, haddock, halibut, lobster, scallop, shrimp, swordfish, tuna, whale
   Beef, pork lamb, chicken
   Cheeses, milk, eggs

MEDICAL AND NUTRITIONAL ROLE

1. **Units:**   1 USP = 1 μg vit. B$_{12}$ = 11,000 LLD units (*L. lactis Dorner* units)

2. **Normal Blood Levels (Man):**   0.08 μg/100 ml (0.03 μg/100 ml, serum)

3. **Recommended Allowances**

   Children—2-5 μg/day
   Adults—5-6 μg/day
   Special—Pregnancy, 8 μg/day; lactation, 6 μg/day; intestinal malabsorption or disease; anorexia; old age; neuropathies; malnutrition; alcoholism

4. **Administration**
   Injection—Parenteral, intramuscular
   Topical—No data
   Oral—Not very effective unless intrinsic factor (enzyme) present

5. **Factors Affecting Availability**
   Decrease
   Cooking losses—Heat labile
   Cobalt deficiency (ruminants)
   Intestinal malabsorption or parasites
   Lack of intrinsic factor
   Intestinal disease, aging
   Vegetarian diet
   Excretion in feces
   Gastrectomy
   Increase
   Administration of sorbitol
   Synthesis by intestinal bacteria (not normally)
   Reduced temperature
   Food in stomach

6. **Deficiency Symptoms**
   Poor growth
   Increased hemolysis of RBC's
   Megaloblastic marrow
   Macrocytic, hyperchromic anemia
   Glossitis
   Degenerative changes in spinal cord, nervous symptoms
   Decreased blood and tissue lipids
   Disturbed carbohydrate metabolism—excretion of methylmalonic acid
   Leukopenia
   Gastrointestinal tract changes
   Loss of hatchability ⎱ Chickens
   Poor feathering   ⎰
   Reproductive failure ⎱ Rats
   Porphyrin whiskers   ⎰
   Dermatitis   ⎱ Pigs
   Impaired reproduction ⎰

7. **Effects of Overdose, Excess**
   Polycythemia reported
   General lack of toxicity

METABOLIC ROLE

1. **Biosynthesis**
   Precursors
      Glycine—corrin nucleus
      δ-Aminolevulinic acid—corrin nucleus
      Methionine—corrin nucleus
   Intermediates
      Porphobilinogen
      α-d-Ribosides of benzimidazole
      5,6-Dimethylbenzimidazole
      α-Ribazole

2. **Production:** Species—Bacteria (some); actinomycetes (some)

3. **Storage:** Liver (30-60%), lungs, kidneys, spleen

4. **Blood Carriers:** α_1-Globulins (52%), α_2-globulins (21%), Albumins (16%), β-globulins (7%), γ-globulins (6%)

5. **Half-life:** > 1 year

6. **Target Tissues:** Central nervous system, kidneys, myocardium, muscle, skin, bone

7. **Reactions**
   Coenzyme forms
      Adenyl cobamide coenzyme (adenyl nucleoside)
      5,6-Dimethylbenzimidazolylcobamide coenzyme
      Benzimidazolylcobamide coenzyme

Organ	Enzyme System	Effect
	MUTASES	
Liver	Glutamate mutase (glut—aspartic)	Activated
Liver	Methylmalonyl CoA mutase (methyl malonic—succinic)	Activated
	DEHYDRASES	
Liver	Diol dehydrase (glycerol-1,3-propanediol)	Activated
Liver	Glycerol dehydrase (glycerol-β-OH-propionaldehyde)	Activated
Liver	Ethanolamine deaminase (ethanolamine-ammonia, acetaldehyde)	Activated

TRANSMETHYLASES

Liver	$B_{1\,2}$ enzyme (homocysteine—methionine) with folate	Activated
Liver	Thymidine synthesis enzymes (purine biosynthesis)	Activated

REDUCTASES

Liver	Methane formation enzymes	Activated
Liver	Ribonucleotide reductase (ribonucleotide— deoxyribonucleotide)	Activated
Liver	Lysine fermentation enzymes	Activated
Liver	Acetate synthesis enzymes	Activated

8. **Mode of Action**
   Cellular
   Anabolic
   DNA synthesis (nucleolar methylations, ribotide conversion)
   RNA synthesis (purine synthesis, nucleolar methylation)
   Protein synthesis (DNA synthesis, methionine synthesis)
   Synthesis of lipids
   Porphyrin synthesis
   Anabolic action—mitosis and growth
   Choline synthesis
   Catabolic
   Carbohydrate metabolism (propionic acid)
   Lipid metabolism (glycerol, ethanolamine)
   Other
   Maintenance of membranes, esp. myelin sheath
   Maintenance of —SH groups in reduced form
   Organismal
   Maintains epithelial and mucosal cells
   Maintains normal bone marrow
   Maintains normal G.I. tract
   Maintains normal CNS
   Maintains erythropoiesis and leukopoiesis
   Maintains body lipids, lipotropic
   Maintains normal growth
   Improves nitrogen retention

9. **Catabolism**
   Intermediates—No body destruction
   Excretion products
   Urine—0.131 μg/day (free)

Feces—34% of ingested dose

Bile—Some reabsorption (enterohepatic recirculation)

MISCELLANEOUS

1. **Relationship to Other Vitamins**

   Folic acid—Active with B$_{12}$ in nucleic acid and methionine synthesis; combined action with vit. B$_{12}$; deficiency of F.A. increases B$_{12}$ absn.

   Vitamin A—Uptake and utilization of carotenes increased with B$_{12}$ in diet; maintenance of mucosal and epithelial cells

   Vitamin B$_6$—Deficiency reduces B$_{12}$ absorption in gut

   Biotin—Active with B$_{12}$ in methylmalonyl CoA metabolism

   Niacin—B$_{12}$ deficiency causes decrease in liver NAD

   Pantothenic acid—B$_{12}$ participates in methylmalonyl CoA conversion; has sparing action of B$_{12}$ and vice versa

   Riboflavin—Possible synthesis from 5,6-dimethylbenzimidazole moiety of B$_{12}$

   Vitamins E, C—Can substitute for vit. B$_{12}$ in certain conditions and synergize it; synergize vit. B$_{12}$ in treatment of macrocytic anemia

   Vitamin B$_1$—Synergistic to B$_{12}$

2. **Relationship to Hormones**

   T4-Deficiency of T4 impairs B$_{12}$ absorption

   Antithyroid antibodies in serum of B$_{12}$ deficient patients

   Increased T4 produces loss of B$_{12}$

   Parathormone—Pernicious anemia found coexisting with hypoparathyroidism (Ca metabolism)

   STH—B$_{12}$ needed for mitosis and growth (with folic acid)

3. **Unusual Features**

   Cyanide group an artifact of preparation

   The only vitamin synthesized in sizable amounts only by microorganisms (possibly in tumors)

   Only vitamin with metal ion

   Works with glutathione

   Glutathione content decreased on B$_{12}$ deficiency

   Mitosis retarded in B$_{12}$ deficiency

   Requires intrinsic factor (enzyme) for oral activity

   Increases tumor size (Rous sarcoma)

   Diamagnetic properties

   No acidic or basic groups revealed on titration (no pKa).

4. **Possible Relationships of Deficiency Symptoms to Metabolic Action**

Degenerative changes in spinal cord—decreased RNA synthesis

Megaloblastic marrow—decreased DNA synthesis (with folate)

Glossitis—decreased cell division of tongue cells

Macrocytic hyperchromic anemia—decreased DNA synthesis of precursor cells

Decreased blood and tissue lipids—possibly due to presence of plasma hemolytic factor in B_{12} deficiency

Disturbed CHO metabolism—activation of methylmalonic acid mutase by B_{12}

Leukopenia—decreased DNA synthesis in stem cells

GI tract changes—decreased cell division of gastric mucosal cells

Increased hemolysis—presence of plasma hemolytic factor in B_{12} deficiency

11
Ascorbic Acid

GENERAL INFORMATION

1. **Synonyms:** Vitamin C, antiscorbutic vitamin, cevitamic acid, hexuronic acid

2. **History**
   1757—Lind described scurvy
   1907—Holst and Frolich produced experimental scurvy
   1928—Zilva described antiscorbutic agents in lemon juice
   1928—Szent-Györgyi isolated hexuronic acid from lemon juice
   1932—Waugh and King identified hexuronic acid as antiscorbutic agent
   1933—Haworth established configuration of hexuronic acid
   1933—Reichstein synthesized hexuronic acid
   1933—Haworth and Szent-Györgyi changed name of hexuronic acid to ascorbic acid

3. **Physiological Forms:** l-Ascorbic acid, dehydroascorbic acid

4. **Active Analogs and Related Compounds:** l-Glucoascorbic acid, d-arabo-ascorbic acid, l-rhamnoascorbic acid, 6-desoxy-l-ascorbic acid

5. **Inactive Analogs and Related Compounds:** d-Ascorbic acid

6. **Antagonists:** d-Glucoascorbic acid, deoxycorticosterone

7. **Synergists:** Vitamins A, E, B_{12}, B_6, K, pantothenic acid, testosterone, STH, folic acid

8. **Physiological Functions**
   Absorption of iron
   Cold tolerance, maintenance of adrenal cortex
   Antioxidant
   Metabolism of tryptophan, phenylalanine, tyrosine
   Growth
   Wound healing
   Synthesis of polysaccharides and collagen
   Formation of cartilage, dentine, bone, teeth
   Maintenance of capillaries

9. **Deficiency Diseases and Disorders:** Scurvy, megaloblastic anemia of infancy

10. **Sources for Species Requiring It:**
    Most species require it (most make it)
    Exogenous sources—Primates, Guinea pig, Indian fruit bat, red vented bulbul, trypanosomes, yeast
    Endogenous sources—Remainder of vertebrates, invertebrates, plants, and some molds and bacteria

CHEMISTRY

1. **Structure**

Ascorbic Acid, $C_6H_8O_6$

2. **Reactions**

Heat—Labile	Oxidation—Labile
Acid—Stable	Reduction—Stable (reducing agent)
Alkali—Labile	Light—Labile
Water—Acid (pH 3) labile	

3. **Properties**
   Appearance—White powder

MW—176.12

MP—190-192°C (decomp.)

Crystal Form—plates, needles

Salts—Ca, Na, metals

Important Groups for activity

    Lactone ring

    Enolic hydroxyls

Solubility

    H_2O—0.3 g/ml

    Acet., Alc.—Slightly sol.

    Benz., Chl., Eth.—Insol.

Absn. Max.—245 mμ (acid)

            265 mμ (neutral)

Redox Potential—E_0^1 = +0.166 volt

    (pH 4)

Chemical Nature—Hexose acid

α_D^{25} = +20.5° H_2O)

Misc.—pKa_1 = 4.17

       pKa_2 = 11.57

4. Commercial Production

Microbiological—*Acetobacter suboxidans* oxidative fermentation of calcium d-gluconate.

Chemical—Oxidation of l-sorbose

5. Isolation

Sources—Adrenal cortex, citrus juices

Method—Ppt. from citrus juice as Pb-complex; crystallize from alcohol-petroleum ether

6. Determination

Bioassay—Guinea pig growth or tooth structure; serum alkaline phosphatase

Physicochemical—Titration against standard oxidizing dye solution, colorimetry of excess dye.

DISTRIBUTION AND SOURCES

1. Occurrence

Plants (High):

    Fruit—Strawberry, citrus, pineapple, guava, black currant, West Indian cherry

    Vegetables—Cabbage, turnip greens, tomatoes, broccoli, kale, horseradish, parsley, corn

    Nuts—English walnuts (green)

    Miscellaneous—Rose hips, molds

Animals: All-Retina > pituitary > corpus luteum > adrenal cortex > thymus > liver > brain > testes > ovaries > spleen > thyroid >

pancreas $>$ saliv. glands $>$ lungs $>$ kidney $>$ intestine $>$ heart
muscle $>$ WBC $>$ RBC $>$ plasma

Microorganisms

No intestinal synthesis except in rat

Produced by certain molds

Required by bacteria, yeasts, and molds for multiplication

2. **Dietary Sources**

High: 100-300 Mg/100 g

Broccoli, brussel sprouts, collards, horseradish, kale, parsley, peppers (sweet), turnip greens

Black currant, guava, rose hips

Medium: 50-100 mg/100 g

Beet greens, cabbages, cauliflower, chives, kohlrabi, mustard, watercress, spinach

Lemons, oranges, papayas, strawberries

Low: 25-50 mg/100 g

Asparagus, lima beans, beet greens, chard, cowpeas, mint, okra, spring onions, peas, potatoes, radishes, rutabagas, turnips, dandelion greens, fennel, soybeans, summer squash

Gooseberries, passion fruit, grapefruit, limes, loganberries, mangoes, cantaloupes, honeydews, red currants, white currants, tangerines, raspberries, tomatoes, kumquats

MEDICAL AND NUTRITIONAL ROLE

1. **Units:**   1 I.U. = 1 U.S.P. unit = 0.05 mg l-ascorbic acid

2. **Normal Blood Levels:**   0.5-1 mg% (plasma), 25 mg% (white blood cells); vary with diet

3. **Recommended Allowances**

Children—40 mg/day

Adults—60 mg/day (males), 55 mg/day (females)

Special—Pregnancy (60 mg/day), lactation (60 mg/day); increased with infection, stress, trauma, allergies, old age, increased protein consumption

4. **Administration**

Injection—Intramuscular, intravenous

Topical—No data

Oral—Preferred route

5. **Factors Affecting Availability**
   Decrease
   　　Damage to adrenal cortex, presence of antagonists
   　　Food preparation (oxidation, storage, leaching, cooking)
   Increase
   　　Storage in body (adrenal cortex)
   　　Antioxidants, synergists in diet

6. **Deficiency Symptoms**
   General
   　　Hyperkeratotic papules on buttocks and calves
   　　Perifollicular hemorrhage, edema
   　　Wound healing failure
   　　Teeth and gum defects
   　　Weakness, listlessness, rough skin, aching joints
   　　Scorbutic bone formation
   Lab animals
   　　Anemia, loss of weight
   　　Abnormal collagen, no intercellular cement

7. **Effects of Overdose**
   None noted—Essentially nontoxic in man, except as noted below
   Possible kidney stones, in gouty individuals
   Inhibitory in excess doses on cellular level (mitosis inhibited)
   Possible damage to β-cells of pancreas and decreased insulin production
   　　by dehydroascorbic acid

METABOLIC ROLE

1. **Biosynthesis**
   Precursors—d-Mannose, d-fructose, glycerol, sucrose, d-glucose, or d-galactose
   Intermediates—UDP glucose, d-glucuronic acid, gulonic acid, l-gulono-lactone, (Mn^{++} cofactor)

2. **Production**—Species and Sites
   All animals (except primates, guinea pig, fruit bat, bulbul)—kidney and liver (rat—intest. bacteria supply)
   Plants (green leaves, fruit skin)
   Cell sites—Microsomes, mitochondria, golgi

3. **Storage Sites:**   Adrenal cortex (small amount)

4. **Blood Carriers:**   Free in blood, especially in white blood cells

5. **Half-life:**   16 days (man), few days (guinea pig)

6. **Target Tissues:**   Adrenal cortex, pituitary, ovary, connective tissue, bone, liver, teeth, gums

7. **Reactions**

Coenzyme form: Redox couple—l-ascorbic ⇌ dehydroascorbic acid

Organ	Enzyme Systems	Effect
	HYDROXYLATING	
Connective tissue	Proline → hydroxyproline (collagen synth.)	Activated
Liver	Tryptophan → 5-hydroxytryptophan (tryptophan metab.)	Activated
Adrenal cortex	Deoxycorticosterone → hydroxy-corticosteroids (steroid hormone synth.)	Activated
	OXIDATION-REDUCTION	
Liver	DPNH—cytochrome b_5 (electron transport)	Activated
Liver	Tyrosine—homogentisic acid (tyrosine metabolism)	Activated
Liver	Glutathione (reduction reaction)	Activated
Liver	Ascorbic acid oxidase (oxidation reactions)	Activated
Liver	Plasma iron—ferritin (reduction)	Activated
Liver	Amidases, proteases, glycosidases, peroxidases, esterases	Activated
Liver	Arginase, papain, liver esterase, catalase, cathepsin	Activated
Liver	Urease, b-amylase	Inhibited

8. **Mode of Action**
   Cellular
   Anabolic
   Collagen synthesis—Proline hydroxylation
   Steroid synthesis—Accelerates acetate incorp. into cholest.
   Serotonin, melanin synthesis
   Polysaccharide synthesis—Chondroitin sulfate incorp.
   Catabolic—Antimitotic agent

Other
Cellular antioxidant—Maintains membranes
Respiration—Cellular reductions and oxidations
Maintenance of electron transport chain in mitochondria
Maintains low redox level for vit. E and sulfhydryl enzymes
Maintenance of peroxidase system (detoxification)
Stimulates phagocytosis
Organismal
Absorption of iron, ferritin production.
Maintenance of adrenals and ovaries (hormone biosynthesis)
Maintenance of connective tissues
Maintenance of steroid endocrine glands
Maintains stress and wound healing reactions
Maintenance of cartilage, bone, and teeth
Maintenance of capillaries, control hemorrhage
Respiration—maintains oxygen turnover

9. **Catabolism**
Intermediates—Diketogulonic acid, oxalic acid
Excretion products
Urine—12-14% excreted as l-ascorbic acid
      12-18% excreted as diketogulonic acid
      24-63% excreted as oxalic acid
Also in feces, sweat, respiratory CO_2.

MISCELLANEOUS

1. **Relationship to Other Vitamins**
Vitamin A—Depletion causes drop in plasma vit. C levels; protected by
    vit. C against oxidation
Vitamin B_{12}—Replaced by vit. C in lactic acid bacteria; can be replaced
    or potentiated by vit. C
Folic acid—Vitamin C decreases symptoms of folic acid deficiency;
    formation promoted by vit. C, stimulates formation of citrovorum
    factor (folinic acid)
Pyridoxine—Pyridoxine-PO_4 and vit. C related to tyrosine metabolism
Vitamin E—Decreased synthesis and excretion of vit. C in vit. E deficient
    animals; protected by vit. C agrainst oxidation
Pantothenic acid—Compensated partly by vit. C in deficiency of
    pantothenic acid

2. Relationship to Hormones

Serotonin—Produced from tryptophan under influence of vit. C

Thyroxine—Cold survival capacity due to vit. C (mediated via thyroxine)

Epinephrine, Norepinephrine—Produced from tyrosine under influence of vit. C; vit. C protects against oxidation

Deoxycorticosterone—Depresses action of vit. C on growth of skeletal tissues

Aldosterone, estradiol-17β, testosterone, cortisol—Vit. C stimulates conversion of deoxycorticosterone in adrenal cortex (maybe needed for steroid synthesis)

Cortisone—Alleviates scorbutic symptoms in joints

STH, ACTH, FSH, LH—High concentrations of vit. C noted in pituitary tissues; STH a synergist in growth

3. Unusual Features

Only d-form active

Antistress factor and anti-infection factor

Activates terminal oxidases in respiratory systems

Sensitivity to oxidation by heavy metals (e.g., Cu) hemochromogens, and quinones

Ease of reversible oxidation

Increased excretion due to barbiturates and drugs

Increased synthesis of vit. C due to chloretone in vit. C deficient animals

Production of H_2O_2 on aerobic oxidation

Increases nitrogen assimilation by plants

Protects tissues against ionizing radiation

4. Possible Relationships of Deficiency Symptoms to Metabolic Action

Failure to produce intercellular cement—Decrease of mucopolysaccharide synthesis from glucuronic acid

Hemorrhage—Weak intercellular fibers causing capillary fragility

Poor tooth and gum structure—Decreased collagen, mucopolysaccharide synthesis; bacterial invasion

Lethargy—Decreased supply of adrenocortical and adrenal hormones

Edema—Decreased aldosterone synthesis and capillary fragility

Weight loss—Possibly decreased growth hormone level

12
Biotin

GENERAL INFORMATION

1. **Synonyms:** Bios IIB, protective factor X, vit. H, egg white injury factor, CoR

2. **History**
   1924—Miller fractionated yeast growth factor Bios into Bios, I, IIB, IIc
   1933—Allison *et al.* isolated CoR (respiratory factor legume nodule bacteria)
   1934—Lease and Parsons described egg white injury in chicks
   1936—Kögl, Tonnis isolated growth stimulant from yeast, and egg yolk, and named it biotin
   1940—György identified vit. H, CoR, and biotin as equivalent
   1941—Williams *et al.* found egg white injury due to antivitamin, avidin (inactivates biotin)
   1942—Du Vigneaud characterized and determined structure of biotin
   1943—Harris synthesized biotin

3. **Physiological Forms**
   d (or +) Biotin (*cis*-form) (β-isomer, *d*(β-biotin)*cis*)
   Of 8 possible stereoisomers (4 *cis*, 4 *trans*), only one active: *d*-biotin (*cis*)
   α and β-isomers based on orientation of isomeric side chains of *cis* and *trans* forms

4. **Active Analogs and Related Compounds**
    Desthiobiotin in some species
    dl-Oxybiotin (microorganisms, rats, chicks)
    Biotinol (in rats)
    Biotin sulfoxide (in some)
    Biocytin (in some)

5. **Inactive Analogs and Related Compounds**
    dl-Epibiotin (*cis*)
    dl-Allobiotin (*trans*)
    dl-Epiallobiotin (*trans*)
    l-Biotin (*cis*)
    α and β-Isomers of these

6. **Antagonists**
    Desthiobiotin in some forms
    Ureylene phenyl
    Homobiotin
    Ureylenecyclohexyl butyric and valeric acids
    Norbiotin
    Avidin
    Lysolecithin
    Biotin sulfone

7. **Synergists:**   Vitamins B_2, B_6, B_{12}, folic acid, pantothenic acid, STH,
    testosterone

8. **Physiological Functions**
    As coenzyme for
    Carboxylation reactions
    Pyruvic oxidase
    Decarboxylation of OAA, succinate, aspartate, malate
    Biosynthesis of aspartate, citrulline, unsaturated fatty acids
    Growth
    Maintenance of skin, hair, sebaceous glands, nerves, bone marrow, sex
    glands

9. **Deficiency Diseases and Disorders (Man)**
    Nonspecific dermatitis
    Seborrheic dermatitis in infants, furunculosis

10. Sources for Species Requiring It

Most organisms require it

Exogenous sources—Most vertebrates, invertebrates, some bacteria and fungi (intestinal bacteria supply needs of man)

Endogenous sources—Higher plants, most fungi and bacteria

CHEMISTRY

1. Structure

$d(\beta\text{-Biotin})(cis)$, $C_{10}H_{16}N_2O_3S$

2. Reactions

Heat—Stable

Acid—Unstable

Alkali—Unstable

Water—Acidic

Oxidation—Unstable

Reduction—Forms desthiobiotin

Light—Stable

3. Properties

Appearance—White powder

MW—244.3

MP—230-32°C

Crystal Form

Orthorhombic (α)

Colorless needles (β)

Salts—Na

Important Groups

Solubility

H_2O—0.03 g/100 ml

Alc.—Sol.

Acet., Benz. Chl. Eth.—Insol.

Absn. Max.—234 mμ

Chemical Nature

Diamino-, monocarboxylic acid

Substituted amino acid

Miscellaneous—pI = 3.5

$\alpha_D^{21} = +91°$ (0.1 N NaOH)

4. **Commercial Production**
    Use meso-diamino succinic acid derivative of fumaric acid for starting
        synthesis

5. **Isolation**
    Sources—Egg yolk, liver, milk
    Method—Extraction with acetone, precipitation with alc. and phospho-
        tungstate, adsorb and elute from charcoal, ppt. with $HgCl_2$,
        dissolve, purify, crystallize

6. **Determination**
    Bioassay
        Microbiological—*L. arabinosus*
        Rat and chick method—Growth response after biotin deficiency
    Physicochemical: Polarography

DISTRIBUTION AND SOURCES

1. **Occurrence**
    Plants
        Fruit—All low
        Vegetables—All low, except beans, peas, cauliflower
        Nuts—All medium, also cereals
    Animals: All low except in organs (esp. liver and kidneys are high)
    Microorganisms: Afford best source of biotin, especially yeast, lower
        fungi and bacteria

2. **Dietary Sources**
    High: 100-400 mg/100 g
        Royal jelly, yeast, lamb liver, pork liver
    Medium: 10-100 mg/100 g
        Wheat, rice, corn, oats, barley
        Eggs, beef liver, chicken, mushrooms
        Cowpeas, chick-peas, lentils, soybeans, cauliflower, chocolate
        Mackerel, salmon, sardines
        Almonds, peanuts, pecans, walnuts, filberts, hazelnuts
    Low: 0-1 mg/100 g
        Cheese, milk
        Apples, bananas, strawberries, cantaloupes, grapefruit, grapes, oranges,
            peaches, watermelon, avocados

Lima beans, beets, carrots, cabbages, corn, lettuce, onions, peas, sweet potatoes, tomatoes, spinach, beet greens
Beef, lamb, veal, pork, tuna, halibut, oyster

MEDICAL AND NUTRITIONAL ROLE

1. **Units:**   By weight, μg

2. **Normal Blood Levels:**   1.23 mg/100 ml (average)

3. **Recommended Allowances**
    Children—Unknown
    Adults—150-300 mg/day estimated. Sufficient supply from intestinal bacteria and diet

4. **Administration**
    Injection—parenteral, intramuscular
    Topical—No data
    Oral—Mainly used

5. **Factors Affecting Availability**
    Decrease
        Presence of avidin in food
        Cooking losses
        Antibiotics
        Sulfa drugs
        Binding in foods (yeast, animals)
    Increase: Synthesis by intestinal bacteria

6. **Deficiency Symptoms**
    General
        Desquamation of the skin
        Lassitude, somnolence, muscle pain
        Hyperesthesia
        Seborrheic dermatitis
    Alopecia, spastic gait, and kangaroo-like posture (rats and mice)
    Dermatitis and perosis (chicks and turkeys)
    Progressive paralysis, K^+ deficiency (dogs)
    Alopecia, spasticity of hind legs (pigs)
    Thinning and depigmentation of hair (monkeys)

7. **Effects of Overdose**
   None noted—1 g/kg not toxic
   Essentially nontoxic in man

METABOLIC ROLE

1. **Biosynthesis**
   Precursors—Pimelic acid, cysteine, carbamyl phosphate
   Intermediates—Desthiobiotin

2. **Production:**   Species and Sites
   Plants—Seedlings, leaves
   Fungi—Some
   Bacteria—Intestinal, some others

3. **Storage Sites:**   Liver

4. **Blood Carriers:**   Unknown

5. **Half-life:**   Requires 3-4 weeks to produce human deficiency with avidin

6. **Target Tissues:**   Skin, nervous tissue, male genitalia, bone marrow, liver, kidney

7. **Reactions**
   Coenzyme forms: CO_2-biotin-enz; d-biotin-lys-enz

Organ	Enzyme System	Effect
	CARBOXYLASES	
Liver	Propionyl-CoA carboxylase	Activated
	β-methylcrotonyl-CoA carboxylase	
	Acetyl-CoA carboxylase	
	Phosphoenolpyruvate carboxykinase	
	ATP-dependent pyruvic carboxylase	
	TRANSCARBOXYLASES	
Liver	Oxalosuccinate-acetyl-CoA transcarboxylase	Activated
	Methylmalonyl-oxalacetic transcarboxylase	
Liver	Malic enzyme	Activated
Liver	Ornithine transcarbamylase	Activated

8. **Mode of Action**

    Cellular

        Anabolic—Purine, protein, and carbohydrate synthesis; synthesis of aspartic acid, oleic acid, fatty acids

        Catabolic—Deamination of serine in animals; tryptophan metabolism

        Other—CO_2 fixation; ureido carbon of enzyme-bound biotin is the "active carbon"; implicated in carbamylation reactions

    Organismal—Growth; maintenance of sebaceous glands, nervous tissue, skin, blood cells, hair, male genitalia

9. **Catabolism**

    Intermediates—Little known

    Excretion products

        Urine—0.4 g/kg/day biotin, biocytin sulfoxide (?)

        Feces—2.5 x amount in food intake (bacterial synthesis)

MISCELLANEOUS

1. **Relationship to Other Vitamins**

    Pantothenic acid—Indicated by depigmentation of hair in deficiency of biotin + pantothenic acid

    Vitamin C—ascorbic acid biosynthesis requires biotin

    Vitamins B_2, B_6, niacin, A, D—Synergistic with biotin in maintenance of skin

    Niacin—Not synthesized from tryptophan in biotin deficiency

    Folic acid—(With pantothenic acid and biotin) increased stress response in adrenalectomized rats

2. **Relationship to Hormones**

    Testosterone—Rat male genital system retarded in biotin deficiency (symptoms develop earlier than in female)

    Cortisol—Adrenocortical insufficiency noted in biotin deficient rats.

    STH—Synergist in growth

3. **Unusual Features**

    Binding and inactivation by avidin protein found in egg white

    Fetal tissues and cancer tissues are higher in biotin than adult tissues

    Biotin deficiency increases severity and duration of some diseases notably some protozoan infections

    Oleic acid and related compounds act to replace biotin as unspecific stimulatory compounds in bacteria

Combines to lysine residues of proteins
Only (+) isomer active
Inactivated by rancid fats, choline

4. **Possible Relationships of Deficiency Symptoms to Metabolic Action**

Desquamation of skin—Decreased fatty acid synthesis, synergism with A, D, other B vitamins

Hyperesthesia—Increased lactic acid levels

Lassitude, somnolence—Decreased oxidation of pyruvate

Muscle pain—Increased lactic acid levels, decreased fatty acid synthesis

Seborrheic dermatitis—Decreased synergism with vits. A, D, other B vitamins

13
Folic Acid

GENERAL INFORMATION

1. Synonyms: Folacin, pteroylmonoglutamic acid, antianemia factor, *L. casei* factor, vit. B_c, vit. M, PGA

2. History
>   1931—Wills demonstrated a factor from yeast active in treating anemia
>   1938—Day *et al.* found yeast or liver extracts active in treating anemia in monkeys
>   1939—Hogan and Parrott prevented anemia in chicks with liver extract
>   1940—Snell and Peterson isolated *L. casei* growth factor from liver and yeast
>   1941—Hutchings *et. al.* found *L. casei* factor also essential for chicks
>   1941—Mitchell, Snell, Williams isolated bacterial (*S. lactis R*) growth factor similar to *L casei* factor from yeast; named it folic acid
>   1943—Stokstad reported *L. casei* factor from liver more active than that from yeast; evidence for multiple factors
>   1946—Angier *et al.* isolated pteroylmonoglutamic acid, proved structure and synthesized it

3. Physiological Forms: Tetrahydrofolic acid, pteroyltriglutamic acid, pteroylheptaglutamic acid, l-folinic acid (citrovorum factor), dihydrofolic acid (5-formyl-5,6,7,8-tetrahydro-PGA) (leucovorin)

4. **Active Analogs and Related Compounds:**   Pteroic acid (bacteria), 10-formyl-FAH_4, 5,10-methenyl-FAH_4, diopterin, 5,10-methylene-FAH_4, 5-formimino-FAH_4, rhizopterin (bact.), xanthopterin (bact.), biopterin (urine), ichthyopterin (fish), leucopterin (invertebrates)

5. **Inactive Analogs and Related Compounds:**   d-folinic acid

6. **Antagonists:**   Aminopterin (4-amino-PGA), methotrexate (amethopterin) pyrimethamine, 4-amino-pteroylaspartic acid

7. **Synergists:**   Biotin, pantothenic acid, niacin, Vits. B_6, B_2 C, B_1, E, B_{12}, STH, estradiol, testosterone

8. **Physiological Functions:**   Synthesis of nucleic acid, coenzyme in purine-pyrimidine metabolism, serine-glycine conversion, intermediate in metabolism of purines and pyrimidines, differentiation of embryonic nervous system, one-carbon transfer mechanisms, metabolism of tyrosine and histidine, formation of active formate, and methionine, synthesis of choline

9. **Deficiency Diseases and Disorders:**   Anemias (macrocytic, megaloblastic, pernicious), glossitis, diarrhea, G.I. lesions, intestinal malabsorption, sprue

10. **Sources for Species Requiring It**
    Most animals require it
    Exogenous sources—Vertebrates, invertebrates, some bacteria (intestinal bacteria provide it in man, rats, dogs, pigs, rabbits) required by monkey, guinea pig, mice, fox, chicken, geese, turkeys
    Endogenous sources—Intestinal bacteria, fungi, yeast

CHEMISTRY

1. Structure

| Pteridine | p-amino-benzoic acid | Glutamic acid |

Folic acid, $C_{19}H_{19}N_7O_6$

2. Reactions

Heat—Labile (in soln.)   Oxidation—Labile
Acid—Labile   Reduction—Stable
Alkali—Stable   Light—Labile (in soln.) to UV
Water—Stable (acid, pH 4.4)

3. Properties

Appearance—yellow crystals   Solubility
MW—441.2 H_2O—0.01 mg/ml
MP—Chars at 250°C   Acet., Alc.—Insol.
Crystal Form—Lenticular   Benz., Chl., Eth.—Insol.
Salts—Ba, Na, Pb   Absn. Max.—282, 350 mμ
Important Groups for activity   (pH 7.0)
  Glutamic acid   Misc.—pK_a = 8.2
  N^{10}, N^5, N^3, N^8 α_D^{25} = ±23° (0.1 N NaOH)
                                Chemical Nature—Purine, amino
                                  acid, benzoic acid

4. Commercial Production

Extraction from yeast or liver; synthetic

5. Isolation

Sources—Spinach, liver, yeast, alfalfa, wheat bran
Method
    Extract (aq.) liver at pH 3.0
    Adsorb on norite, elute with NH_4OH-ethanol

Adsorb on superfiltrol pH 1.3, elute with NH_4OH-ethanol
Ppt. with Ba^{++}, pH 7.0 in alcohol
Esterify with methanol, extract with n-butanol
Adsorb on superfiltrol pH 7, elute ester with 75% acetone
Crystallize from hot methanol, hydrolyze ester
Recrystallize from hot H_2O

6. Determination

Bioassay
  Animal—chick feathering, rat oviduct development
  Microbial—Growth of *L. casei, S. fecalis*
Physicochemical
  Enzymatic—DPNH reductase activity
  Fluorometric—Fluorescence at 470 mμ
  Colorimetric—Estimate aromatic amine on cleavage
  Polarographic—Paper chromatography

DISTRIBUTION AND SOURCES

1. Occurrence

Plants: Fruit—Low
  Vegetables—Green leafy vegetables, dried beans
  Nuts—Almonds, filberts, peanuts, walnuts
  Miscellaneous—Green leaves, grass, barley, oats, rye, wheat
Animals
  Liver, kidney
  Butterflies (wing pigment, xanthopterin)
  Fish scales (ichthyopterin)
Microorganisms: Intestinal bacteria, yeast, fungi, algae
Miscellaneous: Mushrooms

2. Dietary Sources

High: 90-300 mg/g
  Liver (beef, lamb, pork, chicken)
  Asparagus, spinach
  Wheat, bran
  Dry beans (lentils, limas, navy)
  Yeast
Medium: 30—90 mg/100 g
  Kidney (beef)

Lima beans, snap beans, broccoli, corn, beet greens, chicory, endive, kale, parsley, chard, turnip greens, watercress

Almonds, filberts, peanuts, walnuts

Barley, oats, rye, wheat

Low: 0-30 mg/100 g

Beef (muscle, heart), lamb, pork, chicken, turkey (muscle)

All fruit tested

Cheese, milk

Brazil nuts, coconuts, pecans

Wax beans, beets, brussel sprouts, cabbages, carrots, brown rice, cauliflower, celery, cucumbers, eggplant, escarole, mustard, kohlrabi, lettuce, mushrooms, okra, onions, parsnips, peas, peppers, potatoes, pumpkins, radishes, rutabagas, squash, sweet potatoes, tomatoes, turnips

MEDICAL AND NUTRITIONAL ROLE

1. **Units:**   By weight, mg

2. **Normal Blood Levels:**   3.53 μg/100 ml (humans)

3. **Recommended Allowances**
   Children and adults
   0.4 mg/day estimate
   Provided by intestinal synthesis in man
   Required by monkey, guinea pig, mice, fox, chicken, geese, turkeys
   Special—Pregnancy, illness

4. **Administration**
   Injection—subcutaneous
   Topical—No data
   Oral—Preferred route

5. **Factors Affecting Availability**
   Decrease
   High urinary excretion (75% ingested)
   Destruction by certain intestinal bacteria
   Increased urinary excretion caused by vit. C
   Sulfonamides block intestinal synthesis
   Poor absorption

Increase—Intestinal bacterial synthesis and release: man, rats, dogs, pigs, rabbits

6. **Deficiency Symptoms**
    Intestinal disturbances
    Leucopenia
    Glossitis
    Thrombocytopenia
    Macrocytic anemia
    Pernicious anemia
    Sprue
    Megaloblastic erythropoiesis
    Gingivitis, agranulosis (monkey)
    Hydrocephalus, splenic enlargement (rats)
    Endocrine disturbances, poor feathering (chick)
    Lethargy, convulsions (guinea pig)

7. **Effects of Overdose**
    Man—No toxicity reported
    Mice—Renal damage, convulsions: LD_{50} = 600 mg/kg
    Chick—Arrest cells in metaphase with high doses

METABOLIC ROLE

1. **Biosynthesis**
    Precursors: Paraminobenzoic acid, glutamic acid, unknown pteridine
    Intermediates: Paraminobenzoylglutamic acid

2. **Production:**   Species and Sites
    Plants—Leaves, seeds, cereal germ, algae
    Bacteria—Intestinal supply sufficient for man, rats, pigs, dogs, rabbits; Other species require exogenous sources
    Fungi—yeast

3. **Storage:**   Liver (small amount)

4. **Blood Carriers:**   Prefolic acid A

5. **Half-life:**   75% of ingested folic acid excreted in urine in 24 hr

6. **Target Tissues:**   Liver, bone marrow, lymph nodes, kidneys

7. Reactions

Coenzyme forms: Folinic acid (citrovorum factor), 10-formyl-FH_4, 5,10-methylene-FH_4,   5-formimino-FH_4,   10-formimino-FH_4, 5-methyl-FH_4, 5-hydroxymethyl-FH_4

Organ	Enzyme System	Effect
Liver	REDUCTASES Dihydrofolate reductase: $FH_2 \rightarrow FH_4$ N^5N^{10}-Methylene-FH_4 reductase: N^5N^{10}-methylene-$FH_4 \rightarrow N^5$-methyl-FH_4	Activated

Liver	TRANSFERASES
	 Formiminoglutamate formimino transferase:
	     Formation of formimino glutamate
	 Serine transhydroxymethylase: Glycine-serine
	     interconversion
	 Formylglutamate formyl transferase:
	     Formation of glutamate
		Activated

Liver	ISOMERASES N^5-formyl-tetrahydrofolate isomerase: N^5-formyl-$FH_4 \rightarrow N^{10}$-formyl-FH_4	Activated
Liver	SYNTHETASES Formyl tetrahydrofolate synthetase: $FH_4 \rightarrow N^{10}$-formyl-FH_4	Activated
Liver	CONJUGASES Folic acid conjugase: Converts pteroyltriglutamate $\rightarrow$ PGA	Activated

8. Mode of Action

Cellular
   Anabolic
     Purine and pyrimidine synthesis
     Choline synthesis
     Methionine synthesis
     Formation of lignin, nicotine, betaine
   Catabolic—Histidine metabolism, tryptophan metabolism
   Other
     Mitotic step: Metaphase $\rightarrow$ anaphase requires folic acid
     Serine-glycine interconversion
     Formiminoglutamate formation
Organismal
   Erythropoiesis, growth
   Maintenance of sex organs
   Maintenance of intestinal tract

Leukopoiesis
Differentiation of nervous system

9. Catabolism
Intermediates: Xanthopterin, leucopterin
Excretion products: Urine—Biopterin, leucovorin, pteroylglutamic acid, 10.8 μg/day (humans); feces—enterohepatic circulation of folate

MISCELLANEOUS

1. Relationship to Other Vitamins
Vitamin C
Facilitates conversion of folic to folinic acid (CF-citrovorum factor)
Protects folinic acid from oxidation, increases urinary excretion of CF
Fundamental role with folic acid in erythropoiesis
Vitamin B_{12}
Blood and marrow changes in pernicious anemia respond to folic acid or B_{12}
Neurological changes in pernicious anemia involve B_{12} and folic acid
Involved with folic acid in formation of methionine from homocysteine
Biotin—Aids in storage and utilization of pantothenic acid in liver, (with folic acid)
Pantothenic acid—Utilization in CoA synthesis (with biotin and folic acid)
Niacin
Need folic acid for niacin metabolism
DPNH required for production of N^5-methyl-FH_4
DPN involved in methionine formation (with folic acid)
Vitamin B_6—Required with folic acid for serine-glycine transformations and for methionine formation
Riboflavin—Required with DPN, folic acid, vit. B_{12}, vit. B_6, for methionine formation

2. Relationship to Hormones
Estradiol—Folic acid deficiency eliminates normal response of female reproductive organs to estrogens; pregnancies not normal
Testosterone—Folic acid increases action of testosterone on development of accessory sex organs
STH—Synergist in growth

3. **Unusual Features**

    Folic acid antagonists used in cancer therapy with temporary remissions

    Occurs in chromosomes

    Distributed throughout cell

    Needed for mitotic step metaphase $\rightarrow$ anaphase

    Antibody formation decreased in folic acid deficiency

    Choline-sparing effects

    Analgesic in man—pain threshold increased

    Low intravenous toxicity in man

    Antisulfonamide effects

    Enterohepatic circulation of folate

    Synthesized by psittacosis virus

    Concentrated in spinal fluid

4. **Possible Relationships of Deficiency Symptoms to Metabolic Action**

    Cytopenia—Decreased nucleic acid synthesis and porphyrin synthesis

    Intestinal disturbances—Indirect relationship with other vitamin deficiencies

    Thrombocytopenia—Decreased nucleic acid synthesis

    Leukopenia—Decreased nucleic acid synthesis

    Glossitis—Indirect effect of other vit. B deficiencies

    Macrocytic anemia and pernicious anemia—Vitamin B_{12} lack and decreased porphyrin synthesis

    Sprue—Indirect effect of lack of other vitamins

14
Niacin

GENERAL INFORMATION

1. **Synonyms:**   Nicotinic acid, nicotinamide, P-P factor, antipellagra factor, anti-blacktongue factor, B_4

2. **History**
   - 1867—Huber first synthesized nicotinic acid
   - 1914—Funk isolated nicotinic acid from rice polishings
   - 1915—Goldberger demonstrated that pellagra is a nutritional deficiency
   - 1917—Chittenden and Underhill demonstrated that canine blacktongue is similar to pellagra
   - 1935—Warburg and Christian determined niacinamide essential in hydrogen transport as DPN
   - 1936—Euler *et al.* isolated DPN and determined its structure
   - 1937—Elvehjem *et al.* cured blacktongue with niacinamide from liver
   - 1937—Fouts *et al.* cured pellagra with niacinamide
   - 1947—Handley and Bond established conversion of tryptophan to niacin by animal tissues

3. **Physiological Forms:**   Niacinamide, NAD (DPN, CoI), NADP (TPN, CoII), N^1-methylnicotinamide

4. **Active Analogs and Related Compounds:**   Niacin esters, coramine, β-picoline, 3-hydroxymethylpyridine

5. **Inactive Analogs and Related Compounds:**   Trigonelline

6. **Antagonists:**   Pyridine-3-sulfonic   acid   (bacteria),   3-acetylpyridine,
6-aminonicotinamide, 5-thiazole carboxamide

7. **Synergists:**   Vitamins B_1, B_2, B_6, B_{12}, D, pantothenic and folic acids, STH

8. **Physiological Functions:**   Maintenance of NAD, NADP; hydrogen and
electron transfer agents in CHO metabolism; furnish coenzymes for
dehydrogenase systems; coenzyme in lipid catabolism, oxidative
deamination, photosynthesis

9. **Deficiency Diseases, Disorders:**   Pellagra (man), blacktongue (dogs), malnutrition, dermatosis (man)

10. **Sources for Species Requiring It**
Required by all species:
Exogenous sources: Animals, some bacteria and fungi (not available from
intestinal bacteria in man, but some conversion from tryptophan
occurs in tissues)
Endogenous sources: Plants: algae, some bacteria and fungi. Animals:
(some species partly via tryptophan; other species completely via
tryptophan)

CHEMISTRY

1. **Structure**

 Niacin, $C_6 H_5 O_2 N$

2. **Reactions**

Heat—Stable	Oxidation—Stable
Acid—Stable	Reduction—Unstable
Alkali—Stable	Light—Stable
Water—Acidic	

3. **Properties**

Appearance—White crystalline powder	Salts—HCl, metallic, Na
MW—123.1	Important Groups for activity
MP—234-237°C (sublimes)	—N on ring
Crystal Form—needles	—COOH

Solubility	Chemical Nature—Carboxylic
H_2O—1 g/100 ml	acid; amine; substituted
Alc.—Sol.	pyridine
Benz., Chl., Eth., Acet.—Insol.	Misc.—pKa = 4.8, 12.0
Absn. Max.—261.5 mμ	α_D = 0 (inactive)

4. **Commercial Production**
   Hydrolysis of 3-cyanopyridine
   Oxidation of nicotine, quinoline, or collidine

5. **Isolation**
   Sources—Liver, yeast
   Method—Remove lipids with solvents; hydrolyze with acid or alkali;
      extract niacin from acidified hydrolyzate; isolate as an acid, ester,
      or Cu salt; purify by recrystallization or sublimation

6. **Determination**
   Bioassay
      Animal—Dogs, blacktongue (curative)
      Microbial—*L. arabinosus*, growth
   Physicochemical
      Colorimetric—Cyanogen Br + reducing agent → color
      Spectrophotometric—UV max. of DPN, TPN

DISTRIBUTION AND SOURCES

1. **Occurrence**
   Plants:
      Fruit—All low (exc. avocados and dried figs, dates, and prunes—
         medium)
      Vegetables—All low (exc. beans, peas, potatoes, broccoli, asparagus,
         corn, parsley, kale—medium)
      Nuts—All medium (exc. coconuts, pecans—low)
   Animals: All medium [exc. livers, kidneys, beef heart, rabbit, turkey
      and chicken (white meat), tuna, halibut, swordfish—high]
   Microorganisms—All high—intestinal bacteria, some other bacteria

2. **Dietary Sources**
   High: 10,000-100,000 μg/100 g (10-100 mg/100 g)
      Peanuts (roasted), rice bran
      Liver (beef, calf, chicken, pork, sheep)

Heart (calf), kidney (pork, beef)

Rabbit, turkey and chicken (white meat)

Meat extract

Tuna, halibut, swordfish

Yeast

Medium: 1000-10,000 µg/100 g (1-10 mg/100 g)

Avocados, dates (dry), figs (dry), prunes (dry)

Asparagus, beans (kidney, lima, snap, wax), broccoli, corn, kale, lentils (dry), parsley, peas, potatoes, soybeans (dry)

Almonds (dry), cashew nuts, chestnuts, walnuts

Barley, oats, wheat, rye, brown rice, wheat germ, molasses, cheeses (camembert, swiss, roquefort)

Beef, veal, chicken (dark meat), duck, lamb, fish (exc. tuna, halibut, swordfish), clams, shrimp, oysters

Mushrooms

Low: 100-1000 µg/100 g (0.1-1.0 mg/100 g)

Apples, apricots, bananas, berries (black-, blue-, cran-, rasp-, straw-), cherries, currants, figs, grapes, grapefruit, lemons, melons, oranges, peaches, pears, pineapples, plums, raisins (dry), tangerines

Beets, beet greens, brussels sprouts, cabbage, carrots, cauliflower, celery, chicory, endive, cucumbers, dandelion greens, eggplant, kohlrabi, lettuce, onions, parsnips, peppers, pumpkins, radishes, rhubarb, spinach, sweet potatoes, tomatoes, turnips, watercress

Coconuts, pecans

Eggs, milk

MEDICAL AND NUTRITIONAL ROLE

1. **Units**—By weight, mg equivalents

2. **Normal Blood Levels:** 0.42-0.84 mg/100 ml

3. **Recommended Allowances**

Children—8-15 mg equivalents/day*

Adults—18 mg equivalents/day—male*; 13 mg equivalents/day—female*

Special—Pregnancy, 15 mg equivalents/day; lactation, 20 mg equivalents/day

---

* Depends on tryptophan content of diet; allow 10 mg equivalents for each 600 mg dietary tryptophan; assume 60 g/day protein in diet has 600 mg tryptophan.

4. **Administration**
   Injection—I.V.
   Topical—No data
   Oral—Preferred route

5. **Factors Affecting Availability**
   Decrease
      Cooking losses
      Bound form in corn, greens, seeds, partially unavailable
      Oral antibiotics
      Decreased absorption—disease
      Decreased tryptophan converted in B_6 deficiency
   Increase
      Alkali treatment of cereals
      Storage in liver, possibly muscle, kidney
      Increased intestinal synthesis

6. **Deficiency Symptoms**
   General (man)—Pellagra
      Retarded growth, achlorhydria
      Weakness, anorexia, indigestion, lassitude, dermatitis, pigmentation, diarrhea, tongue erythema, irritability, headaches, insomnia, memory loss
   Histological changes in CNS (dog, cat—blacktongue)
   Drooling (dog, cat—blacktongue)
   Perosis (chickens)
   Poor feathering (chickens)

7. **Effects of Overdose**
   Man—Limited toxicity starting approx. 1-4 g/kg dosage with individual variations in sensitivity. Burning, itching skin, peripheral vasodilation, decreased serum cholesterol, fatty liver, stimulated CNS, increased (pulse rate, respiratory rate, cerebral blood flow), decreased blood pressure
   Rat—Respiratory paralysis, ketosis
   Dogs—Death
   Chick—Inhibition of growth, fatty liver

METABOLIC ROLE

1. **Biosynthesis**

    Precursors—Tryptophan (animals, bacteria). Glycerol and succinic acid (plants)

    Intermediates—Kynurenine, hydroxyanthranilic acid, quinolinic acid

2. **Production:**   Species and Sites

    Fungi—*Neurospora*

    Plants—Leaves, germinating seeds, shoots

    Bacteria—Intestinal

    Animals—Tissues (not intestinal)

3. **Storage:**   Liver, heart, muscle

4. **Blood Carriers:**   Mostly as DPN in blood corpuscles

5. **Half-life**—1/3 of intake excreted in 24 hr

6. **Target Tissues:**   Liver (storage), heart, muscle, kidney, skin, G.I. tract, spinal cord

7. **Reactions**

    Coenzyme forms—(DPN,NAD) and (TPN,NADP). Act as redox couples: oxid $\leftrightharpoons$ reduced)

Organ	Enzyme System	Effect
	More than 50 metabolic reactions known	
Liver	DEHYDROGENASES: Alcohol, lactate, malate, isocitrate, glucose-6-P-succinic, β-hydroxy-butyrate, 3β-hydroxysteroids, betaine aldehyde, glutamate, α-glycerophosphate, uridine DPG, reduced glutathione, glyceraldehyde-3-P	Activated
Liver	OXIDASES: α-keto glutaric oxidase microsomal mixed function oxidases (DPN + TPN), oxidation of steroids, fatty acids, drugs and carcinogens	Activated or completed

8. **Mode of Action**

    Cellular

    Anabolic—Maintains microsomal reductive biosynthesis; photosynthesis

Catabolic
Furnishes coenzymes for lipid catabolism
Oxidative deamination
CHO metabolism—Dehydrogenation, oxidation
Key reactions in glycolysis, TCA cycle, and HMP
Other
Hydrogen and electron transfer agent
A mobile hydrogen transfer agent
Maintains respiratory chain in mitochondria
Organismal
Maintains growth
Maintains energy supply to organism from degradation of carbo-
hydrates, proteins, and lipids
Maintains terminal section of respiratory cycle
Maintains manufacture of hormones (steroids) proteins, lipids
Stimulates gastric secretion and bile secretion

9. **Catabolism**
Intermediates—N^1-Methylnicotinamide (liver)
Excretion Products
Feces: Nicotinic acid
Urine: N^1-Methylnicotinamide; N^1-methyl-6-pyridone-3-carboxamide

MISCELLANEOUS

1. **Relationship to Other Vitamins**
Vitamin B_2—Flavo-proteins reoxidize NAD, NADP
Vitamin B_6—Decreased tryptophan conversion to niacin in B_6 deficiency
Vitamins B_1, B_2, B_6, Pantothenic Acid, Folic Acid, Vitamin B_{12}—
General synergism with niacin in alleviating deficiencies and in CHO
metabolism
Vitamins B_1, B_2, B_6—Needed for conversion of tryptophan to niacin

2. **Relationship to Hormones**
Serotonin—Reduces tryptophan conversion to niacin (in cancer cases)
Thyroxine, Insulin—Affect mitochondrial metabolism (as do DPN and
TPN), and energy production from CHO metabolism
Cortisol, Testosterone, Estradiol, Progesterone, Aldosterone—DPN and
TPN involved in steroid oxidations in liver, in steroid hormone
synthesis, and in cholesterol metabolism
STH—Synergist in growth

3. **Unusual Features**

Has hormonal quality, being partially internally synthesized

Vasodilator, causes flushing (not as niacinamide)

High corn diets cause deficiency due to tryptophan deficiency in corn
protein and unavailability of niacin in corn

Prepared from nicotine using strong oxidizing agent

Stereospecific action of dehydrogenases on DPN

Serum cholesterol lowering with large doses

Antagonist (6-aminonicotinamide) active against some rat tumors

Other pyridine derivatives functional in DPN and TPN

Conversion of tryptophan not in intestines

Toxicity of overdose preventable by feeding methionine (rats)

4. **Possible Relationships of Deficiency Symptoms to Metabolic Action**

Retarded growth—General synergism of all B vitamins

Dermatitis, itching, pigmentation, tongue lesions; other B vitamins, esp.
B_2, involved

Irritability, mental disturbances, nervous lesions related to thiamine
synergism with niacin

G.I. lesions and disturbances related to thiamine deficiency and
synergism

Mottled liver, fatty liver are disturbances of cholesterol metabolism

15
Pantothenic Acid

GENERAL INFORMATION

1. Synonyms: Chick antidermatitis factor, B3, Bios IIa, antigray-hair factor

2. History
   1901—Wildiers described Bios, essential for yeast growth
   1933—Williams isolated crystalline Bios from yeast; named it panto-
       thenic acid
   1938—Williams isolated pantothenic acid from liver
   1939—Jukes determined liver antidermatitis factor (chick) identical to
       yeast factor
   1939—Woolley *et al.* demonstrated β-alanine a vital part
   1940—Harris, Folkers, *et al.* reported structure determination and
       synthesis of pantothenic acid; crystallization also
   1950—Lipmann *et al.* discovered CoA
   1951—Lynen characterized coenzyme A structure

3. Physiological Forms: Coenzyme A, pantotheine, d(+)pantothenic acid

4. Active Analogs and Related Compounds: Pantothenyl alcohol, β-alanine
       (bacteria), pantotheine (LBF), pantothine, pantothenylcystine,
       ethylmonoacetylpantothenate, ethyl pantothenate

5. Inactive Analogs and Related Compounds: l-pantothenate, α-alanine
       analogs

6. **Antagonists:** Pantoyltaurine, ω-methylpantothenic acid, bis(β-pantoyl-aminoethyl)disulfide, 6-mercaptopurine, pantoylaminoethanethiol

7. **Synergists:** Biotin, folic acid, vit. C, B_{12}, B_1, B_2, niacin, STH

8. **Physiological Functions:** Part of coenzyme A in carbohydrate metabolism (2 carbon transfer-acetate, or pyruvate), lipid metabolism (biosynthesis and catabolism of fatty acids, sterols, + phospholipids), protein metabolism (acetylations of amines & amino acids), porphyrin metabolism, acetylcholine production, isoprene production

9. **Deficiency Diseases, Disorders:** Dermatitis (chick), achromotrichia (rat), adrenal necrosis (rats), bloody whiskers (rat), alopecia (mice)

10. **Sources for Species Requiring It**
    All organisms require it
    Endogenous sources—Higher plants
    Exogenous sources—All other organisms (not available from intestinal synthesis in man)

CHEMISTRY

1. **Structure**

d(+)-Pantothenic acid, $C_9H_{17}O_5N$

Pantoic acid β-Alanine

2. **Reactions**

Heat—Labile	Oxidation—Stable
Acid—Labile (warm)	Reduction—Stable
Alkali—Labile (warm)	Light—No data
Water—Sol. (acid)	

3. **Properties**

Appearance—yellow viscous oil	MP—unstable
MW—219.24	Crystal Form—No data

Salts—Calcium, sodium
Important Groups for activity
β-amino group
Solubility
H_2O—7 g/100 ml
Acet., Alc.—Sol.
Benz., Chl., Eth.—Insol.

Absn. Max.—358 mμ
Chem. Nature—Conjugated amino
acid, polyhydroxy acid
Miscellaneous:
$\alpha_D^{25} = (+37.5°)$ (H_2O)
pKa = 4.4

4. **Commercial Production:**   Synthetic
Condensation of d-pantolactone with salt of β-alanine

5. **Isolation**
Sources—Rice, bran, liver, yeast
Method
Extract liver with 90% ethyl alc.
Adsorb out organic bases on Fuller's earth
Adsorb vitamin on charcoal, pH 3.6, elute with ammonia
Form brucine salts, extract selectively with $CHCl_3$
Convert brucine salt to calcium salt
Purify by fractional ppt. from organic solvents

6. **Determination**
Bioassay
Animal—Growth rate of chicks
Microbiol—Growth of *L. casei*
Physicochemical—Estimate of β-alanine after hydrolysis; estimate CoA
by citrate cleavage enzyme

DISTRIBUTION AND SOURCES

1. **Occurrence**
Plants
Fruit—All (low)
Vegetables—All (medium and low)
Nuts—All (high and low)
Animals
All (medium and high)
Organs (brain, heart, kidney, liver)
Microorganisms
Yeast (high), Rumen bacteria in sheep and cattle
Molds

2. **Dietary Sources**

High: 2.0 mg-10.0 mg/100 g

Beef (brain, heart, liver, kidney), pork (liver, kidney), sheep liver, chicken liver, lamb kidney

Eggs

Herring, cod ovary

Wheat germ, bran, dried peas, peanuts

Yeast, royal jelly

Medium: 0.5 mg-2.0 mg/100 g

Salmon, clams, mackerel

Walnuts

Broccoli, soybeans, oats, lima beans, cauliflower, peas, avocado, carrots, kale, dried lentils, spinach, rice

Beef, pork (ham, bacon), chicken, lamb

Mushrooms, wheat, cheese

Low: 0.1-0.5 mg/100 g

Bananas, oranges, peaches, pears, pineapples, tomatoes, apples, grapes, grapefruit, lemons, plums

Onions, kidney beans, cabbage, lettuce, peppers, white and sweet potatoes, turnips, watercress

Almonds

Oysters, lobster, shrimp

Veal

Milk, honey, molasses

MEDICAL AND NUTRITIONAL ROLE

1. **Units:** By weight, mg

2. **Normal Blood Levels:** 19-32 μg/100 ml

3. **Recommended Allowances**
   Children—no data
   Adults—Exact values unknown, estimate 10-15 mg/day
   Special—Increased needs in stress situations

4. **Administration**
   Injection—Parenteral
   Topical—No data
   Oral—Preferred route

5. **Factors Affecting Availability**
    Decrease
        Cooking—Up to 44% loss
        Heat instability
        Difficult release of bound forms
    Increase: Intestinal bacteria synthesis (very little in man)

6. **Deficiency Symptoms**
    General
        Neuromotor disturbances
        Cardiovascular disorders
        Digestive disorders
        Infection susceptibility
        Physical weakness, depression
    Stress susceptibility—rats
    Skin disorders (cornea)—rats, chicks
    Liver disorder—rat, chick
    Reproductive failure—chick
    Decreased antibody production—rat

7. **Effects of Overdose**
    10 g/kg in mice, respiratory failure
    Essentially nontoxic in man

METABOLIC ROLE

1. **Biosynthesis**
    Precursors
        α-Ketoisovaleric acid (pantoic acid)
        Uracil (β-alanine)
        Aspartic acid (β-alanine)
    Intermediates
        Ketopantoic cid
        Pantoic acid
        β-alanine

2. **Production: Species and Sites**
    Plants—Green plants, fungi
    Bacteria—Intestinal

3. **Storage:**   Possibly liver, heart, kidney (all small amounts)

4. **Blood Carriers:**   Blood proteins

5. **Half-life:**   Estimate average loss: 25% of daily requirements

6. **Target tissues:**   All, esp. brain, heart, kidney, liver

7. **Reactions**

   Coenzyme form: CoA (adenine -3'-P-Ribose-P-P-pantothenic acid-β-mercapto ethylamine)

Organ	Enzyme System	Effect
Liver	TRANSFERASE: Citrate condensing enzyme β-Ketothiolase, CoA transferase	Activated
Brain	TRANSACYLASES: Choline acetylase, lipoic transacetylase, phosphotransacetylase	Activated
Liver	ISOMERASES: Methylmalonyl isomerase, β-hydroxyacyl racemase, enoyl isomerase	Activated
Liver	ESTERASES: Acetyl CoA deacylase, succinyl CoA deacylase	Activated
Liver	HYDRASES: Enoylhydrase	Activated
Liver	SYNTHETASES: Acetic thiokinase, fatty acid thiokinases, succinic thiokinase, acetyl carboxylase, propionyl carboxylase, methyl crotonylcarboxylase	Activated
Muscle and liver	DEHYDROGENASES: Hydroxyacyldehydrogenase, pyruvate dehydrogenase, α-ketoglutarate dehydrogenase acyl dehydrogenases	Activated

8. **Mode of Action**

   Cellular

   Anabolic

   Lipid synthesis increased

   Active in synthesis of porphyrins, acetylcholine and isoprenoid groups

   Sterol and hormone synthesis increased

   Catabolic—Regulates CHO metabolism

   Other—As coenzyme A in CHO, lipid, and protein metabolism. Acyl transfer agent.

   Organismal

   Fat synthesis and breakdown

   Respiratory pigment synthesis

   Water metabolism regulator

   Energy metabolism regulator

9. Catabolism
> Intermediates—Not destroyed in body
> Excretion Products
>> Urine—Pantothenic acid (1-7 mg/day)
>> Feces—Variable

MISCELLANEOUS

1. Relationship to Other Vitamins
> Folic acid—Required for utilization of pantothenic acid
> Biotin—Required for utilization of pantothenic acid; acts with pantothenic acid in fatty acid biosynthesis; reduces severity of pantothenic acid deficiency in rats
> Vitamin C—Compensates partly for deficiency of pantothenic acid
> CoQ—Decreased in pantothenic acid deficiency
> Vitamin A and Vitamin E—Synthesis promoted by pantothenic acid (isoprene production)
> Pantothenic acid and biotin involved in synthesis of niacin

2. Relationship to Hormones
> Aldosterone, Deoxycorticosterone, Cortisol, Testosterone, Progesterone—Cholesterol precursors for sterol hormones in adrenal cortex require pantothenic acid for synthesis; pantothenic acid deficiency produces cortical necrosis
> Cortisone—Relieves certain pantothenic acid deficiency symptoms in humans
> STH—Produces pantothenic acid deficiency in rats; synergist in growth

3. Unusual Features
> Promotes amino acid uptake
> Anticarcinogenic agent (?) (A. E. Needham)
> Potentiated by Zn in preventing graying of hair in rats
> Resistance to stress of cold immersion
> Deficiency of pantothenic acid in tumors
> Chick hatchability depends on pantothenic acid
> Useful in treating vertigo, postoperative shock, poisoning with isoniazid and curare
> Useful in acceleration of wound healing
> Useful in treating Addison's disease, liver cirrhosis, and diabetes

4. **Possible Relationships of Deficiency Symptoms to Metabolic Action**

 Neuromotor Disturbances

 Decreased phospholipid and acetylcholine synthesis

 Has effect on membranes, degeneration of nerves

 Cardiovascular disorders—Disturbances of fat and CHO metabolism due to degeneration of liver

 Digestive disorders—Decreased bile acid production due to decreased sterol production; atrophy of intestinal mucosa

 Infection susceptibility—Decreased antibody production due to decreased ATP synthesis

 Physical weakness and depression—Decreased ATP synthesis

16
Hypothalamic-Releasing Factors

CORTICOTROP(H)IN-RELEASING HORMONE (CRH)

1. **Synonyms:** CRF, cortical-releasing factor (hormone), (adreno) corti-cotrop(h)in-releasing factor

2. **History**
   1955—Saffran *et al.* first demonstrated release of ACTH by crude hypothalamic extract
   1962—Schally *et al.* proposed structure for CRH
   1963—Critchlow *et al.* reported CRH preparation maintains ACTH synthesis in pituitary transplants

3. **Forms:** α_1, α_2, and β

4. **Analogs:** Vasopressin, oxytocin

5. **Functions:** Chemical stimulant; messenger from hypothalamus to ACTH-producing cells in anterior pituitary; stimulates production of ACTH

6. **Structure**
   Peptide with disulfide ring system
   α_1—16 amino acids, similar to α-MSH
   α_2—13 amino acids, almost identical to α-MSH
   β—11 amino acids, similar to arginine vasopressin

7. MW—Approx. 1100 (β), 1500 (α)

8. **Extraction; Purification:**   Acid acetone, pH 1.5, ppt. with $(NH_4)_2SO_4$, chromatography, countercurrent distribution

9. **Determination**
    Bioassay—Release of corticosteroids in rat plasma on injection of CRH

10. **Factors Affecting Release of CRH**
    Stimulators—Stress, low level of cortisol, sympathomimetic amines
    Inhibitors—Cerebral cortex factors

11. **Production Sites and Storage Location**
    Hypothalamus—Ventral area, neurohypophysis

12. **Target Tissues:**   Anterior pituitary (ACTH-producing cells)

13. **Reactive Intermediate:**   Cyclic AMP

14. **Unusual Features:**   Very unstable

LUTEINIZING HORMONE-RELEASING HORMONE (LRH)

1. **Synonyms:**   LRF, LH-releasing factor (hormone)

2. **History**
    1941—Guillemin first postulated existence of LH-releasing factor
    1964—McCann and Ramirez caused depletion of ovarian ascorbic acid
        with extracts of hypothalamus
    1964—Campbell *et al.* infused hypothalamic extract into anterior
        pituitary and produced ovulation

3. **Functions:**   Chemical stimulant: messenger from hypothalamus to LH-producing cells in anterior pituitary

4. **Structure:**   Peptide containing Asp., Glu., Gly., Ala., Lys., His., Arg., Thr., Prol., Leu., Ser.

5. MW—1200-2500

6. **Extraction; Purification:**   Acetic acid extraction; gel filtration on sephadex G-25, chromatography

7. **Determination:**   Bioassay—Depletion of ovarian vit. C

8. **Factors Affecting Release of LRH**
    Stimulators—Low levels of estradiol, testosterone, norepinephrine, cate-
        cholamines
    Inhibitors—High levels of LH, testosterone

9. **Production Sites and Storage Location:**   Hypothalamus

10. **Target Tissues:**   Anterior pituitary (LH-producing cells)

11. **Reactive Intermediate:**   Cyclic AMP

THYROTROP(H)IN-RELEASING HORMONE (TRH)

1. **Synonyms:**   TRF, TSH-releasing factor (hormone)

2. **Antagonists:**   T3, T4 (large doses)

3. **History**
    1958—Harris and Woods produced thyroidal I_{131} release on stimulation
        of hypothalamus
    1958—Nikitovich *et al.* produced TSH after reimplanting pituitary graft
        near median eminence, but not in temporal lobe area
    1969—Byler *et al.* determined structure of porcine TRH

4. **Functions:**   Chemical stimulant: messenger from hypothalamus to TSH-
        producing cells in anterior pituitary

5. **Structure:**   Porcine TRH: Tripeptide
    L-pyroglutamyl—L-histidyl—L-proline amide

6. **MW:**   Approx. 400

7. **Extraction: Purification:**   Gel filtration; high-voltage electrophoresis

8. **Factors Affecting Release of TRH**
    Stimulators—Low level of T4, cold, stress, light, Ca^{++} ion
    Inhibitors—No data

9. **Production Sites and Storage Location:**   Suprachiasmatic area, median
        eminence, neurohypophysis

10. **Target Tissue:**   Anterior pituitary (TSH-producing cells)

11. **Reactive Intermediate:**   Cyclic AMP

12. **Unusual Properties:**   Destroyed in human serum in 15 min at 37°C

FOLLICLE STIMULATING HORMONE-RELEASING HORMONE (FRH)

1. **Synonyms:**   FSH-RF, FSH-releasing factor (hormone), FRF, FSH-RH

2. **History**
   - 1932—Hollweg and Junkmann proposed CNS involved in secretion of gonadotropins
   - 1964—Igarishi *et al.* demonstrated FSH-releasing activity of hypothalamic extracts
   - 1964—Mittler and Meites demonstrated FRH increases release of FSH in pituitary culture

3. **Functions:**   Chemical stimulant: messenger from hypothalamus to FSH-producing cells in anterior pituitary

4. **Structure:**   Polyamine, MW = < 300

5. **Extraction: Purification:**   Similar to LRH, plus long columns of sephadex G-25.

6. **Factors Affecting Release of FRH**
   Stimulators—Estrogen level (cyclic), K^+ ion
   Inhibitors—Stress, FSH

7. **Production Sites and Storage Location:**   Median eminence

8. **Target Tissues:**   Anterior pituitary (FSH-producing cells)

9. **Reactive Intermediate:**   Cyclic AMP

PROLACTIN RELEASE-INHIBITING HORMONE (PIH)

1. **Synonyms:**   PIF, RIH, prolactin inhibiting factor (hormone)

2. **History**

    1963—Meites showed increased prolactin secretion by pituitaries in tissue culture while other hormones decreased

    1962-63—Talwalker; Basteels *et al.* reduced prolactin in pituitary culture by adding hypothalamic extract

3. **Functions:** Chemical inhibitor: messenger from hypothalamus to prolactin-producing cells in anterior pituitary

4. **Structure:** Some similarity to LRH, probably a peptide

5. **Extraction: Purification:** 0.1 N HCl extract, concentrate and separate on sephadex G-25

6. **Factors Affecting Release of PIH**

    Stimulator—Prolactin

    Inhibitor—Reserpine

7. **Production Sites and Storage Location:** Satiety center, appetite suppressor in hypothalamus

8. **Target Tissues:** Prolactin-producing cells in anterior pituitary

9. **Reactive Forms:** No data

10. **Unusual Features:** Stable to boiling

GROWTH HORMONE-RELEASING HORMONE (GRH)

1. **Synonyms:** GRF, somatotrop(h)in-releasing factor (hormone), growth-hormone-releasing factor (hormone), SRF, GHRF

2. **History**

    1964—Deuben and Meites released GH in rat pituitary in tissue culture using rat hypothalamic extracts

    1965—Schally *et al.* stimulated release of GH by incubating rat pituitaries with beef, pig, hypothalamic extracts

3. **Functions:** Chemical stimulant; messenger from hypothalamus to STH-producing cells in anterior pituitary

4. **Structure:**   Acidic polypeptide

5. **MW:**   2500 (approx.)

6. **Extraction: Purification:**   0.1 N HCl extraction; gel filtration, CMC chromatography

7. **Factors Affecting Release of GRH**
   Stimulators—No data
   Inhibitors—No data

8. **Production Sites and Storage Location:**   Hypothalamus, neurohypophysis

9. **Target Tissues:**   Anterior pituitary cells producing STH

10. **Reactive Intermediate:**   Cyclic AMP

PROLACTIN-RELEASING HORMONE (PRH)

1. **Synonyms:**   PRF, prolactin-releasing factor (hormone)

2. **History**
   1965—Kragt and Meites increased prolactin release in pigeon pituitary culture by pigeon hypothalamic extracts

3. **Functions:**   Stimulates release of prolactin from anterior pituitary (probably only in birds)

4. **Structure:**   Not obtained pure

5. **Extraction: Purification:**   No data

6. **Factors Affecting Release of PRH**
   Stimulators—No data
   Inhibitors—No data

7. **Production Sites and Storage Location:**   Hypothalamus of birds

8. **Target Tissues:**   Anterior pituitary cells secreting prolactin

MELANOCYTE STIMULATING HORMONE RELEASE-INHIBITING HORMONE (MIH)

1. **Synonyms:**   MIF, MSH-inhibiting factor (hormone), MRIH

2. **History**
     1962—Etkin produced frog blackening by repositioning pituitary in other locations in body
     1964—Kastin and Ross produced coloration in albino rat by repositioning pituitary

3. **Functions:**   Inhibits release of MSH from intermediate lobe of pituitary

4. **Structure:**   Not obtained pure

5. **Extraction: Purification:**   2 N acetic acid extraction; gel filtration on sephadex G-25

6. **Factors Affecting Release of MIH**
     Stimulators—No data
     Inhibitors—No data

7. **Production Sites and Storage Location:**   Hypothalamus (paraventricular nucleus)

8. **Target Tissues:**   Cells of intermediate pituitary lobe secreting MSH

MELANOCYTE STIMULATING HORMONE-RELEASING HORMONE (MRH)

1. **Synonyms:**   MRH, MSH-releasing factor (hormone)

2. **History**
     1965—Taliesnik and Orios found evidence for existence of MRH

3. **Functions:**   Stimulates release of MSH from intermediate lobe of pituitary

4. **Structure:**   Not obtained pure

5. **Extraction: Purification:**   No data

6. **Factors Affecting Release of MRH**
   Stimulators: No data
   Inhibitors: No data

7. **Production Sites and Storage Location:**   No data

8. **Target Tissues:**   Cells of intermediate pituitary lobe secreting MSH

17
Growth
Hormone

GENERAL INFORMATION

1. Synonyms: Somatotrop(h)in, GH, STH, phyone, (anterior) pituitary growth hormone, adenohypophyseal growth hormone, somatotrophic hormone, hypophyseal growth hormone

2. History
1921—Evans and Long induced growth in rats with pituitary extract
1930—Smith restored growth in hypophysectomized rats with hypophyseal implants
1945—Li *et al.* isolated growth hormone from anterior pituitary (beef)
1962—Reisfeld *et al.* isolated growth hormone from human anterior pituitary
1964—Glick, Roth, Berson, and Yalow developed accurate immunoassay of growth hormone in serum
1966—Li *et al.* determined amino acid sequence for human growth hormone, 188 amino acid residues
1971—Li *et al.* synthesized human growth hormone

3. Physiological Forms: "Sulfation factor"

4. Active Analogs and Related Forms: Prolactin (human). Chorionic factor

5. Inactive Analogs and Related Forms: Primate GH minus 10% A.A. residues, bovine GH minus 25% A.A.'s, human GH minus C-terminal phenylalanine

6. **Antagonists:** Cortisone, cortisol, insulin (all concentration dependent), plasma inhibitors

7. **Synergists:** Adrenal corticoids (fat metabolism), ACTH, T4, insulin, testosterone

8. **Physiological Functions**
   General growth of organism
   Promotes skeletal growth, protein anabolism, fat metabolism, CHO metabolism, water and salt metabolism

9. **Deficiency Diseases and Disorders**
   Deficiency—Progeria, pituitary dwarf, hypopituitarism
   Excess—Acromegaly, gigantism

10. **Essentiality for Life:** Absence results in stunted, abnormal growth, with possible decrease in normal lifespan

CHEMISTRY

1. **Structure**—Growth hormone, structure known and synthesized (Human)
   Human—Coiled, unbranched protein, 188 A.A. residues, 2S-S-bridges
   (Phe ———— Phe)
   Bovine—Coiled, 1-branch protein, 400 A.A. residues, 4S-S-bridges

   $$\begin{array}{c} Phe \text{--} \\ \end{array} \!\!\!\! \searrow Phe$$
   Phe⁻⁻⌝
   Ala⁻⁻⌟> Phe

2. **Reactions**

   Heat—Stable to $100°C$ 15 min

   Acid—Unstable (strong)

   Alkali—Unstable (strong)

   Water—Soluble, acidic

   Oxidation—Oxidizes S—S bonds

   Reduction—Reduces S—S bonds

   Light—No data

   Proteolysis—15% limit of digestion of human growth hormone before loses activity

3. **Properties**

   Appearance—No data

   MW—21,500 (human)
   48,000 (bovine)

   MP—None

   Crystal Form—None

   Salts—None

   Important Groups for activity
   —S—S—; Phe (terminal)

   Solubility
   H_2O—Sol.
   Acet. Alc.—Insol.
   Benz., Chl., Eth.—Insol.

   Absn. Max.—Approx. 280 mμ

   Chemical Nature—Simple protein, globulin

   Misc- pI = 4.9 (human)
   = 6.8 (bovine)

4. **Commercial Production:**   Not available

5. **Isolation**
   Sources—Pituitary glands of sheep, ox, pig, monkey
   Methods
      Extract with borate buffer, pH 8.8, DEAE chromatography
      Ppt. with $(NH_4)_2 SO_4$, column chromatog. $IRC_5 O$, pH 5.1
      Treat with acetic acid-acet., ppt. with acet.; column chromatog., ppt.
        with alc.
   Additional purification: Counter-current distribution and gel filtration

6. **Determination**
   Bioassay
      Tibia test (rat) (5 μg-120 μg)
      Increased weight (rat)
      Increased N retention (rat)
      S^{35} incorporation into cartilage (rat)
   Physicochemical
   Immunoassay
   Radioimmunoassay

MEDICAL AND BIOLOGICAL ROLE

1. **Species Occurrence, Specificity and Antigenicity**
   Occurrence—All vertebrates except birds
   Specificity—No crossing of species lines for primates or guinea pigs.
      Other vertebrates slightly more tolerant
   Antigenicity—Monkey, sheep, rat, pig hormones antigenically different.

2. **Units:**   1 USP unit = 1 I.U. = 1 mg

3. **Normal Blood Levels:**   20-50 μg/100 ml serum (man)

4. **Administration**
   Injection—Preferred route
   Topical—Not used
   Oral—Not used, inactivated

5. **Factors Affecting Release**
   Inhibitors—Inadequate dietary protein, sleeplessness, hyperglycemia
   Stimulators—Plasma amino acids, hypoglycemia, GHRH, vasopressin
      (fish), adequate protein in diet, fasting, exercise, sleep

6. **Deficiency Symptoms**
   Humans
   　Dwarfism
   　Failure of long bones to close
   　Failure of sexual maturation
   　Increased fat deposition

7. **Effects of Overdose, Excess**
   　Tumors, β-cell destruction
   　Pituitary giants
   　Bone thickening

METABOLIC ROLE

1. **Biosynthesis**
   　Precursors—Amino acids. All 20 standard
   　Intermediates—Unknown
   　Site(s) in Cell—Unknown

2. **Production Sites:**　Anterior pituitary acidophils

3. **Storage Areas:**　Anterior pituitary

4. **Blood Carriers:**　α_2-Macroglobulin, β-lipoprotein

5. **Half-life:** 20 min

6. **Target Tissues:**　All except nervous tissue, esp. bone, viscera, muscle, epiphyseal cartilage

7. **Reactions**
   　Reactive form—Sulfation factor (?)

Organ	Enzyme System	Effect
Most tissues and organs	RNA-polymerase	Activated
	Protein-synthetic	Activated
Blood cells	Alk. phosphatase	Activated

8. **Mode of Action**
   　Cellular
   　　Anabolic
   　　　Increases rate of protein and RNA synthesis
   　　　Increases glycogen deposition (muscles)

Catabolic—Mobilizes unsaturated fatty acids
Other—Increases amino acid permeability of cells; increases salt and H_2O
transport in kidney
Organismal
Increases muscle, skin, viscera, lymph glands, bone and cartilage size
Decreases urea formation
Increases blood sugar
Increases tissue nitrogen
Mobilizes fatty acids from adipose tissue

9. **Catabolism**

Intermediates—Liver destruction, to peptides; plasmin in blood inactivates GH
Excretion Products—Small amounts of GH in urine

MISCELLANEOUS

1. **Relationship to Vitamins**

All vitamins—All concerned with growth

2. **Relationship to Other Hormones**

Insulin—Inhibited by GH in certain concentrations. Synergist with GH at
other (low) concentrations
GHR—GH-releasing factor of hypothalamus
Vasopressin—A hypothalamic release factor (in fish)
Cortisol—Antagonist to GH (protein metabolism). Also a synergist (fat
metabolism)
Testosterone—Synergist with GH
T4—Synergist with GH (differentiation)
ACTH—Synergist with GH

3. **Unusual Features**

Rat GH lacks tryptophan; contaminated with protease
Lactogenic and growth activity present in human GH
Guinea pig not sensitive to own GH
HGH withstands 15 min at 100°C
Increases capacity to form tumors
Lactogenic action in humans, similarity in structure to prolactin

4. Possible Relationships of Deficiency Symptoms to Metabolic Action

Dwarfism—Lack of protein synthesis due to lack of GH activity

Failure of long bones to close—Lack of major metabolic action of GH

Failure of sexual maturation—Lack of synergism of sex hormones and GH

Increased fat deposition—Lack of catabolic action of GH

18
Thyroid-Stimulating Hormone (TSH)

GENERAL INFORMATION

1. **Synonyms:** Thyroid-stimulating hormone, thyr(e)otrop(h)ic hormone, TTH, thyrotrop(h)in

2. **History**

    1921—Evans and Long first noted effects of pituitary extracts on growth

    1927-30—Smith reported that hypophysectomy in rat causes atrophy of thyroids (and other organs) correctable by hypophyseal implants

    1929—Basset; Aron and Loeb defined properties of a thyrotrophic hormone

    1945—Ciereszko isolated crude TSH from beef pituitaries

    1960—Wynston *et al.* obtained purified TSH from beef, sheep, and whale pituitaries

    1963—Carsten *et al.* determined amino acid composition of beef TSH

3. **Physiological Forms:** Unknown

4. **Active Analogs and Related Compounds:** LATS (long-acting thyroid stimulator)

5. **Inactive Analogs and Related Compounds:** TSH minus CHO moeity, oxidized TSH

6. **Antagonists:** Acetylated TSH, *p*-aminosalicylic acid, perchlorate, sulfathiazole, thiocyanate, thiouracil, thiourea

7. **Synergists:** STH, ACTH, MSH, TH

8. **Physiological Functions**

Regulation of body temperature via T4
Maintains thyroid gland and its secretory activity (colloid discharge)
Maintains iodine uptake by thyroid gland
Promotes differentiation in embryo during development (via T4)
Stimulates coupling of diiodotyrosine to form thyroxine (T4)

9. **Deficiency Diseases, Disorders**

Thyrotoxicosis (excess), goiter (excess or deficiency), exophthalmos (excess), Sheehan's syndrome (deficiency)

10. **Essentiality for Life:** Required by all vertebrates for proper development; possible shortening of lifespan in absence of TSH

CHEMISTRY

1. **Structure**

Glycoprotein—Unpurified (contaminated with LH). Contains 2.5% CHO—Glucosamine, galactosamine, hexose, fucose

2. **Reactions**

Heat—Inactivates
Acid—Easily inactivates
Alkali—Inactivates
Water Basic

Oxidation—Inactivates using bromine, iodine, and permanganate
Reduction—May potentiate effects of TSH
Light—No data
Proteolysis—inactivates with pepsin or trypsin

3. **Properties**

Appearance—No data
MW—26-30,000 (300 amino acids)
MP—No data
Crystal Form—No data
Salts—No data
Important Groups for activity
  α-NH$_2$, tyrosine, CHO moiety
  —S—S—

Solubility
  H$_2$O—Sol.
  Acet., Alc.—Insol.
  Benz., Chl., Eth.—Insol.
Absn. Max.—Approx 280 mμ
Chemical Nature—Basic glycoprotein, globulin
MISC—pl = 7·8

4. **Commercial Production:**   Extract bovine pituitary glands

5. **Isolation**
>   Sources—Bovine pituitary glands
>   Methods
>>   Extract pituitary (freeze, dried) in 2% NaCl, pH 7.6. Precipitate at pI
>>   with acetone (1 I.U./mg)
>>   Precipitate from 3.6 M ammonium sulfate
>   Purification
>>   Chromatog. on IRC-50, elute with 1 M NaCl
>>   Chromatog. on CM cell, elute with 0.2 M NaCl 0.05 M formate, pH
>>   3-4
>>   Gel filtration on sephadex G-50, G-100
>>   Chromatog. on IRC-50 in urea (60 I.U./mg)

6. **Determination**
>   Bioassay
>>   Height of secretory epithelium in thyroid—guinea pig
>>   Number colloid droplets in guinea pig thyroid
>> I_2 depletion of 1-day chick
>>   Uptake I^{131} by thyroid of rats
>>   In vitro assay, slice uptake of I^{131}
>   Physicochemical—Radioimmunoassay

MEDICAL AND BIOLOGICAL ROLE

1. **Species Occurrence, Specificity, and Antigenicity**
>   Occurrence—All vertebrates
>   Specificity—Incomplete; bovine TSH active in all species
>>   (chick and guinea pig most sensitive)
>   Antigenicity—High; bovine TSH antigenic in rabbits

2. **Units:**   1 I.U. = 13.5 mg of standard = 1 USP unit

3. **Normal Blood Levels (Man):**   5-20 milliunits/100 ml plasma

4. **Administration**
>   Injection—Preferred route
>   Topical—Inactive
>   Oral—Inactive

5. **Factors Affecting Release**
> Inhibitors
>> Feedback via hypothalamus from high serum T4
>> High serum iodide, massive doses vit. A
>> High temperature
>> Inhibition of hypothalamus
>> Nerve stimuli
>
> Stimulators
>> Release factor of hypothalamus (TRH)
>> Decreased serum T4 via hypothalamus
>> Low temperature
>> Stimulation of hypothalamus
>> Nerve stimuli

6. **Deficiency Symptoms**
> Decreased synthesis of thyroid hormones
> Low serum protein-bound iodine (PBI)
> Decreased iodine uptake by thyroid
> Secondary symptoms of thyroxine deficiency

7. **Effects of Overdose, Excess**
> Exophthalmic effect
> Increased synthesis of thyroid hormones
> Increased PBI
> Increased iodide uptake by thyroid
> Increased basal metabolic rate
> Decreased thyroid iodine
> Decreased blood cholesterol
> Goiter

METABOLIC ROLE

1. **Biosynthesis**
> Precursors—17 of 20 standard amino acids. No glutamine, asparagine, tryptophan
> Intermediates—Unknown
> Site(s) in cell—Basophilic cytoplasm

2. **Production Sites:** S^2 type cell, anterior pituitary

3. **Storage Areas:**   Not stored

4. **Blood Carriers:** β-globulins

5. **Half-life:**   54 min

6. **Target Tissues:**   Thyroid, reproductive glands, liver, probably muscles

7. **Reactions**
    Reactive intermediate—Cyclic AMP (secondary messenger)

Organ	Enzyme System	Effect
Thyroid	Proteolytic enzymes (on colloid)	Activated
Thyroid	Synthetic enzymes for T4	Activated
Thyroid	Adenyl cyclase	Activated
Thyroid	DPN kinase	Activated
Thyroid	HMP enzymes	Activated

8. **Mode of Action**
    Cellular
        Anabolic
            RNA and protein synthesis (thyroid)
            Thyroid hormone synthesis (thyroid)
        Catabolic
            Lipolytic activity increased
            Proteolytic activity increased (thyroid)
            Glucose oxidation increased via TCA, HMP, and glycolysis
        Other
            Activates thyroid cell membrane enzymes
            Increases oxidase granules (thyroid), and O_2 consumption by
                thyroid cells
            Increases glucose and iodine entry into cells
            No increase in $NADP^+$
    Organismal
        Mobilization of thyroid hormones
        Increases serum bound iodine
        Maintains body temperature via T4

9. **Catabolism**
    Intermediates—Hydrolyzed in liver
    Excretion products—Present in urine

MISCELLANEOUS

1. Relationship to Vitamins

Vitamin A—Massive doses of vit. A inhibit secretion of TSH; thyroid hormones required for carotene and retinene conversions

Vitamins B_1, B_2, B_{12}, C—Requirements increased in hyperthyroidism; tissue concentrations reduced

Vitamin B_6, Niacin—Conversion to phosphorylated reactive forms impaired in hyperthyroidism

Vitamins A, D, E, K—Requirements increased in hyperthyroidism; tissue concentrations reduced in hyperthyroidism

2. Relationship to Other Hormones

T4—TSH stimulates production of T4; synergist in lactation

LH—Contained frequently as a contaminant in TSH

3. Unusual Features

Not inactivated by neuraminidase

CHO moiety needed for activity

Different functions in lower species

Rapid loss of potency in solution

Inactivation by freeze drying

Reduction may potentiate activity

High cystine content

Phospholipase activity of TSH reported

4. Possible Relationships of Deficiency Symptoms to Metabolic Action

Decreased synthesis of thyroid hormones—Insufficient activation of thyroid cell membrane enzymes

Low serum PBI—Reduction of T4 output due to decreased TSH

Decreased iodide uptake by thyroid—Decreased reactivity of thyroid gland

19
Follicle-Stimulating Hormone (FSH)

GENERAL INFORMATION

1. **Synonyms:** Follotropin, Luteoantine, Thylakentrin, Prolan A, gonadotropin I, gametogenic hormone, follicle ripening hormone, gametokinetic hormone

2. **History**
   1921—Evans and Long first noted gonadotropic effect of pituitary extracts on rats
   1927-30—Smith reported that hypophysectomy in rat causes atrophy of gonads (and other organs) correctable by hypophyseal implants
   1928—Aschheim and Zondek discovered a follicle-stimulating gonadotropin in menopausal urine
   1933—Fevold *et al.* identified a separate follicle-stimulating hormone in the pituitary
   1939—Chow *et al.* demonstrated FSH to be resistant to inactivation by proteolytic enzymes
   1940—Fevold *et al.* ⎫ Described isolation procedures
   1949—Li, Simpson and Evans ⎭ for animal FSH
   1965—Roos and Gemzell prepared human FSH from menopausal urine

3. **Physiological Forms:** Unknown

4. **Active Analogs and Related Forms:** PMSG, HMG (mixture of FSH and LH)

5. **Inactive Analogs and Related Forms:**   FSH without sialic acid moiety

6. **Antagonists:**   No data

7. **Synergists:**   LH, STH, T4

8. **Physiological Functions:**   Gametogenic
    Female—Stimulates ovarian follicles to grow and to develop, forming multiple layers and antra
    Male—Stimulates seminiferous tubules; stimulates spermatogenesis

9. **Deficiency Diseases, Disorders:**   Klinefelter's syndrome (deficiency), Turner's syndrome (deficiency), hypogonadotropic eunochoidism (deficiency)

10. **Essentiality for Life:**   Not required for life of organism, but required for reproduction by all vertebrates analyzed

CHEMISTRY

1. **Structure:**   Unknown
    Glycoprotein—7.4% sialic acid; impure preparations (contam. with LH) 0.6% hexosamine; 1.3% hexose

2. **Reactions**

    Heat—No data
    Acid—Stable
    Alkali—Stable
    Water—Acidic

    Oxidation—H_2O_2, periodate
        —inactivate
    Reduction—Cysteine,
        ketene—inactivate
    Light—No data
    Proteolysis—Inactivates on 60-75% digestion with trypsin
    Urea—Stable in 6 M urea

3. **Properties**

    Appearance—No data
    MW—30,000 (pig)
        28,000 (sheep)
    MP—No data
    Crystal Form—No data
    Salts—No data

    Important Groups for activity
        Sialic acid (complex CHO)
        —S—S—, terminal NH_2
    Solubility
        H_2O—soluble
        Acet., Alc.—Insol.
        Sol. 50% Acet.

Sol. 70% Alc.   Misc—pl = 5.1 (pig)
Benz., Chl., Eth.—Insol.   = 4.5 (sheep)
Absn. Max.—Approx 280 mμ
Chemical Nature—Acidic
glycoprotein

4. **Commercial Production:**   Extracted from human and sheep pituitaries

5. **Isolation**
   Sources—Human, horse, sheep, swine pituitary
   Method—Extract frozen pituitaries in aqueous salts; fractional precipitation from ammonium sulfate; DEAE cellulose; sephadex G-100; polyacrylamide gel electrophoresis

6. **Determination**
   Bioassay—Problems with LH contamination
     Ovarian weight change
     Stimulation of young ovarian follicles (rabbit)
     Increase in weight of testes
   Physiochemical
     Immunoassay
     Radioimmunassay

MEDICAL AND BIOLOGICAL ROLE

1. **Species, Occurrence, Specificity, and Antigenicity**
   Occurrence—Found in all species of vertebrates studied
   Specificity—Strong species specificity (Fish FSH inactive in mammals)
   Antigenicity—Moderately antigenic

2. **Units:**   1 I.U. = 38.5 μg sheep FSH (NIH—S_1, Std.)

3. **Normal Blood Levels (Man):**   Males: 0.02 I.U./100 ml plasma, females 0.015 I.U./100 ml plasma (Menopausal female: 0.20 I.U./100 ml plasma)

4. **Administration**
   Injection—Preferred route
   Topical—inactive
   Oral—inactive

5. **Factors Affecting Release**

Inhibitors—Estradiol, cortisol, stress, hyperthyroidism, feedback by sex hormones via hypothalamus

Stimulators—FRH from hypothalamus, castration, menopause, low sex hormone levels, female—rhythmic control by hypothalamus via FRH secretion, male—continuous secretion of FRH by hypothalamus

6. **Deficiency Symptoms**

Decreased gametogenic function and development (nonfunctional)

Atrophy of gonads

No maturation of ova, sperm

Obesity

Decreased libido, potency, hair growth

Decreased blood levels of estrogen

7. **Effects of Overdose, Excess**

Hypertrophy of secondary sex organs

Increased growth and maturation of numerous follicles

Increased estrogen secretion (with LH)

Follicular cysts

METABOLIC ROLE

1. **Biosynthesis**

Precursors—All 20 standard amino acids except methionine

Intermediates—Unknown

2. **Production Sites:**   Anterior pituitary—basophilic cells (peripheral)

3. **Storage Areas:**   Anterior pituitary

4. **Blood Carriers:** α, β-plasma proteins

5. **Half-Life:**   Approx. 1 hr

6. **Target Tissues:**   Ovary, testis

7. **Reactions**

Reactive Form—Unknown

Enzyme Systems—Unknown

8. Mode of Action

  Cellular

    Anabolic—Unknown

    Catabolic—Unknown

    Other—Stimulates incorporation of glucose and α-aminoisobutyric acid into rat ovaries

  Organismal

    Promotes growth of ovarian follicles

    Promotes development of ovarian follicle

    Promotes growth of seminiferous tubules

    Promotes spermatogenesis

9. Catabolism

  Intermediates—Liver hydrolysis

  Excretion Products—Free in urine (active)—small amounts

MISCELLANEOUS

1. Relationship to Vitamins

  Vitamin C—Depletion in ovary due to LH and FSH action

  Vitamin E—Needed for maintenance of membranes in sex organs

2. Relationship to Other Hormones

  STH, LH—Synergists to FSH

  PMSG, HMG—Active analogs to FSH

  ACTH—Inhibitor of FSH

  T4—Inhibitor of FSH

3. Unusual Features

  Increased instability with purer preparations

  Only pituitary hormone not precipitated with 50% saturated $(NH_4)_2SO_4$

  Bird migration, ovulation, sex behavior controlled by FSH via light and temperature

  Gonadotropins of mammals stimulate thyroids of fish

  CHO groups needed for activity—neuraminidase inactivates

  Cyclic release in females (spontaneous ovulators)

4. Possible Relationships of Deficiency Symptoms to Metabolic Action

  Decreased gametogenesis and development of gonads, atrophy of gonads, no maturation of ova or sperm, decreased potency—lack of FSH function (unknown)

Obesity—Unknown
Decreased libido—decreased synergism with testosterone and LH
Decreased hair growth—decreased synergism with sex hormones and LH
Decreased blood levels of estrogen—decreased synergism with LH

20
Luteinizing
Hormone (LH)

GENERAL INFORMATION

1. **Synonyms:** Luteotrop(h)in, interstitial cell-stimulating hormone, ICSH, Prolan B, gonadotrop(h)in II, Metakentrin, corpus luteum-ripening hormone

2. **History**

   1921—Evans and Long first noted gonadotropic effect of pituitary extracts on rats.

   1927-30—Smith noted hypophysectomy in rat caused atrophy of gonads (and other organs) correctable by hypophyseal implants

   1933—Fevold *et al.* identified a separate luteinizing hormone in pituitaries

   1940—Li, Simpson, and Evans isolated LH from sheep pituitaries

   1940—Shedlovsky *et al.* ⎫
   1942—Chow *et al.* ⎬ Isolated LH from pig pituitaries

   1962—Squire *et al.* isolated a purified LH from human pituitaries

3. **Physiological Forms:** α and β-forms

4. **Active Analogs and Related Compounds**
   HCG, HMG (mixture of FSH and LH)
   PMSG (properties of FSH and LH)

5. **Inactive Analogs and Related Compounds:** LH minus CHO moiety

6. **Antagonists:**   Prolactin, insulin (both concentration dependent)

7. **Synergists:**   FSH, prolactin, TH, insulin

8. **Physiological Functions**
   Female
      Promotes estrogen and progesterone secretion, ovulation, maintains ovarian tissues
      Stimulates rupture of follicles and formation of corpora lutea
   Male
      Stimulates Leydig cells to secrete testosterone, gametogenic with FSH
      Promotes growth of seminal tubules and accessory sex organs

9. **Deficiency Diseases, Disorders:**   Hypogonadism; irregular sexual development

10. **Essentiality for Life:**   Not required for life of organism, but required for reproduction by all analyzed vertebrates

CHEMISTRY

1. **Structure**
   Globular glycoprotein with S–S bridges (2-5% CHO)
   Ser-Val-Asp–––human
   Ser-Val-Phe–––Ser-Lys (porcine)

2. **Reactions**
   Heat—Inactivates
   Acid—Picric, TCA, picrolonic, and flavianic acids ppt. LH without loss of activity
   Alkali—No data
   Water—Sol., acidic

   Oxidation—H_2O_2, periodate, performic acid—inactivate
   Reduction—Cysteine, ketene—inactivate
   Light—No data
   Proteolysis—Inactivates
   Urea—Unstable in 6 M urea

3. **Properties**
   Appearance—White powder
   MW—26,000 (human)
        30,000 (sheep)
   MP—No data
   Crystal Form—No data

   Salts—No data
   Important Groups for activity
      Cys., Pro.
      CHO moiety
      —S–S—

Solubility
  H_2O—soluble
  Alc.—Sol. 4% alc.,
  Acet., Benz., Chl., Eth.—Insol.
Absn. Max.—Approx 280 mμ

Chemical Nature—Acidic, globular
  glycoprotein
Misc—pI = 5.4 (human)
  = 7.3 (sheep)
  = 7.45 (pig)

4. Commercial Production: Extraction of human or sheep pituitaries

5. Isolation
  Sources—Pituitary of human, sheep, swine, and beef
  Method
    Aqueous extract at pH 5.5
    Ammonium sulfate precipitation
    Metaphosphoric acid precipitation
    Ethanol fractionation
    IRC-50; sephadex G-100

6. Determination
  Bioassay
    Vitamin C depletion of rat ovary
    Increased hyperemia in immature rat ovary
    Increased weight in male sex accessory organs
    Weaver-Finch test
    Physicochemical—Radioimmunoassay

MEDICAL AND BIOLOGICAL ROLE

1. Species Occurrence, Specificity, and Antigenicity
  Occurrence—Found in all vertebrate species studied
  Specificity—Slight species specificity
  Antigenicity—Definite

2. Units: 1 I.U. = 0.67 μg ovine LH (NIH—S_1, Std.)

3. Normal Blood Levels (Man):   1.5-3.0 I.U./100 ml plasma (males and females) preovulatory and menopausal women 7.5-15.0 I.U./100 ml plasma

4. Administration
  Injection—Preferred route
  Topical—Inactive
  Oral—Inactive

5. **Factors Affecting Release**
    Inhibitors
      Cortisol
      Stress
      High sex hormone levels
      Feedback to hypothalamus by sex hormones
      Hyperthyroidism
    Stimulators
      Low sex hormone levels
      External stimuli
      Male—Continuous LRH from hypothalamus
      Female—Continuous LRH (hypothalamus) in induced ovulators—rabbit
      Cyclic LRH (hypothalamus) in spontaneous ovulators—human and dog

6. **Deficiency Symptoms**
    Estrogen or androgen secretion inhibited
    Atrophy of interstitial tissue in ovary or testis
    Lack of ovulation, luteinization in female

7. **Effects of Overdose, Excess**
    Hypertrophy, then atrophy of Leydig cells in male
    Increases estrogen or androgen secretion (with FSH)
    Precocious ovulation and luteinization of prepared follicles

METABOLIC ROLE

1. **Biosynthesis**
    Precursors—19 of 20 standard amino acids, tryptophan missing
    Intermediates—Unknown

2. **Production Sites:**   Anterior pituitary, central cells, basophilic cells

3. **Storage Areas:**   Stored in pituitary prior to ovulation in female

4. **Blood Carriers:**   Complex with inactive protein

5. **Half-life:**   Approx. 1 hr

6. **Target Tissues:**   Gonads

7. Reactions
Reactive intermediate—Cyclic AMP (secondary messenger)

Organ	Enzyme System	Effect
Gonads	Adenyl cyclase	Activated
	Enzymes incorporating acetate into squalene	Activated

8. Mode of Action
Cellular
Anabolic—Increased synthesis of steroid hormones
Female—Interstitial ovarian cells synthesize estradiol
Male—Leydig cells synthesize testosterone
Catabolic—Increased CHO catabolism to produce NADH, NADP
Organismal
Promotes gametogenesis
Promotes growth of accessory sex organs
Stimulates rupture of follicles in ovary

9. Catabolism
Intermediates—Hydrolysis in liver
Excretion products—Active hormone in urine

MISCELLANEOUS

1. Relationship to Vitamins
Vitamin C—Ovarian depletion on LH stimulation
Vitamin E—Involved in spermatogenesis

2. Relationship to Other Hormones
FSH—Synergist to LH
Prolactin—Synergist to LH
HMG—Mixture of FSH and LH
PMSG—Properties of FSH and LH
HCG—Analog to LH

3. Unusual Features
More stable on freeze-drying than FSH
LH causes multiple ovulation in birds
Insensitive to neuraminidase
Inactivated by trypsin and carboxypeptidase, pepsin, chymotrypsin

Not inactivated by CHO splitting enzymes; CHO moiety unharmed

CHO moiety needed for activity

Cyclic release in certain females (spontaneous ovulators)

4. **Possible Relationships of Deficiency Symptoms to Metabolic Action**

Estrogen or androgen secretion inhibited—lack of cyclic AMP to stimulate ovary or testis production

Atrophy of interstitial tissue in ovary or testis—lack of stimulus by cyclic AMP

Lack of ovulation or luteinization in female—lack of cyclic AMP to initiate events leading to ovulation

21
Prolactin

GENERAL INFORMATION

1. **Synonyms:** Lactogenic hormone, luteotrop(h)ic hormone, LTH, luteotrop(h)in, lactogen, galactin, mammotropin

2. **History:**
   1928—Stricker and Grüter discovered prolactin
   1933—Riddle *et al.* coined term prolactin
   1937—Lyons isolated prolactin from pituitary glands of ox, sheep, and pig
   1939—Astwood, Fevold suggested luteotropin distinct from LH
   1941—Evans, Simpson, Lyons suggested identity of prolactin and luteotropin in rat
   1942—Li crystallized prolactin (first pituitary hormone to be crystallized)
   1967—Sherwood showed chemical similarity of human growth hormone to placental lactogenic hormone

3. **Physiological Forms:** In man, prolactin is a part of very pure growth hormone complex

4. **Active Analogs and Related Forms:** 50% digested residue—"active core"

5. **Inactive Analogs and Related Forms**
   Reduced molecule (with cysteine)
   Acetylated molecule—(on lysine residues)
   Iodinated molecule—(tyrosine residues iodinated)

6. **Antagonists:**   Progesterone, testosterone, estradiol, LH (all concentration dependent)

7. **Synergists:**   STH, T4, prednisone, estradiol, progesterone, cortisol, oxytocin, PTH, LH

8. **Physiological Functions**
   Initiation of lactation
   Development of mammary glands in female
   Increases weight and growth (similar to somatotropin) (some species)
   Nidation of zygote
   Protein anabolism (some species)
   Growth and secretion of crop gland (birds)
   Luteotropic (only in mouse and rat)
   Promotes maternal behavior

9. **Deficiency Diseases, Disorders:**   Mammary carcinoma, galactorrhea, failure of lactation

10. **Essentiality for Life:**   Not essential except where it functions as a growth hormone in certain species (birds, reptiles)

CHEMISTRY

1. **Structure**
   Single chain protein, 205 amino acids
   Pig: Ala.———Cys—Tyr—Leu—Asn—Cys
   Sheep: Thre.———Cys—Tyr—Leu—Asn—Cys

2. **Reactions**

Heat—Stable	Oxidation—Inactivates
Acid—Ppt. with 0.5% TCA	Reduction—Inactivates
Alkali—Unstable	Light—Not reported
Water—Soluble, acidic	Proteolysis: 50% digestion leaves active core

3. **Properties**

Appearance—Crystalline powder	Salts—Not reported
MW—25,000 (pig)	Important Groups for activity
23,300 (sheep)	Tyr
MP—Not reported	Lys
Crystal Form—Not reported	Cys (S—S bridges)

Solubility:

  H_2O—Slightly soluble

  Alc.—Sol.

  Acet., Benz., Chl., Ether—Insol.

  Absn. Max.—Approx. 280 mμ

Chemical Nature—Single chain simple acidic protein

$\alpha_D^{25} = -40.5°$ (H_2O)

Misc—pl = 4.97 (pig)

      = 5.74 (sheep)

4. Commercial Production

Extraction of pituitary glands of ox, sheep, swine

5. Isolation

Sources—Pituitary glands of sheep

Methods

  Ovine acetone powder extracted with pH 3 buffer

  Precipitate prolactin with 0.06 saturated NaCl

  Fractional precipitation, pH 5.6

  Probability of protease contamination

Purify by: Countercurrent distribution. DEAE chromatography

6. Determination

Bioassay

  Crop sac thickening (pigeons)

  Mammary gland growth in pseudopregnant rabbit

  Luteotropic, inhibition of estrus (mice)

Physicochemical Assay

  Immunoassay

  Radioimmunoassay

MEDICAL AND BIOLOGICAL ROLE

1. Species Occurrence, Specificity, and Antigenicity

Occurrence—Found in all vertebrates

Specificity—Some tolerance in crossing species lines

Antigenicity—Moderate; bovine X rabbit no antigenicity

2. Units: 1 I.U. = 0.1 mg international standard

3. Normal Blood Levels (Man)

Not detectable in male or nonlactating female

Detectable in lactating women

4. **Administration**
   Injection—Currently used
   Topical—Not active
   Oral—Not active

5. **Factors Affecting Release**
   Inhibitors—Hypothalamus (PIH factor), CNS, progesterone
   Stimulators—CNS, suckling stimulus, oxytocin, tranquilizers, PRH (in birds)

6. **Deficiency Symptoms**
   Lactation not maintained
   Growth inhibited (some species)

7. **Effects of Overdose, Excess**
   Corpus luteum maintained past normal regression time
   Precocious lactation

METABOLIC ROLE

1. **Biosynthesis**
   Precursors—Amino acids, 20 standard
   Intermediates—Unknown
   Site(s) in cell—Not reported

2. **Production Sites**
   Anterior pituitary—acidophils, E cells
   Placenta

3. **Storage Areas:**   Pituitary

4. **Blood Carriers:**   Free and combined with blood proteins

5. **Half-life:**   Unknown

6. **Target Tissues:**   Mammary gland, ovary, crop sac (pigeons)

7. **Reactions**
   Reactive form—Unknown
   Enzyme systems—Unknown

8. **Mode of Action**
   Cellular
   Anabolic—Protein synthesis (some species)
   Catabolic—Unknown
   Other—Unknown
   Organismal
   Initiates and maintains lactation
   Increases life of corpus luteum
   Increases weight and growth
   Releases progesterone (in mouse and rat)

9. **Catabolism**
   Intermediates—Unknown
   Excretion Products—Free in urine; also breakdown products

MISCELLANEOUS

1. **Relationship to Vitamins:** None specifically; all indirectly via growth action in species where applicable

2. **Relationship to Other Hormones**
   Progesterone, STH, T4, PTH, Estradiol, Cortisol, Oxytocin—Synergists with prolactin [STH, prolactin, ACTH (or adrenal steroids) needed for lactation in rats]

3. **Unusual Features**
   Not stimulated, but is inhibited, by hypothalamus (PIH) (except in birds)
   Only anterior pituitary hormone precipitated with 0.5% TCA
   Present in male pituitary (human) and probably in blood of male
   Human prolactin not separated from HGH
   HGH stimulates pigeon crop, lactogenic activity in rabbits + luteotrophic activity in mouse
   New plumage stimulated in birds by prolactin.
   Antigonadal in male bird; otherwise no known functions in male
   Terminal ring similar to oxytocin ring structure
   Different functions in various species

4. **Possible Relationships of Deficiency Symptoms to Metabolic Action**
   Lactation not maintained—Metabolic functions of prolactin absent
   Growth inhibited—Prolactin needed to synergise growth hormone in certain species

22
Adrenocortico-tropic Hormone (ACTH)

GENERAL INFORMATION

1. **Synonyms:** Adrenocorticotrop(h)in, corticotrop(h)ic hormone, adrenocorticotrop(h)ic hormone

2. **History**

    1930—Smith, P. E., first observed direct relationship between the pituitary and the adrenal cortex

    1933—Collip *et al.*; Evans; Houssay *et al.* noted that cell-free extracts of anterior pituitary stimulate adrenal cortex of hypophysectomized animal

    1943—Li *et al.*; Sayers *et al.* isolated from anterior pituitary, protein hormones that stimulate adrenal cortex

    1954—Bell analyzed amino acid sequence of ACTH

    1961—Hofmann ⎫
    1963—Li ⎭ Synthesized ACTH

3. **Physiological Forms:** A_2 (high MW); A_1 (low MW)

4. **Active Analogs and Related Compounds**

    ACTH sequence 1-21 (100% active)

    ACTH sequence 1-20 (30% active)

    ACTH sequence 1-19 with substitutions on #1, 11, 18 (>100% active as ACTH)

    β-Lipotropin (sheep, pig, beef)

5. **Inactive Analogs and Related Compounds:** α-MSH, β-MSH, ACTH sequence 2-39

6. **Antagonists:** Insulin; concentration dependent for corticosterone, cortisol; STH (protein metabolism)

7. **Synergists:** Epinephrine, cortisol, corticosterone, STH (fat metabolism)

8. **Physiological Functions**
   Maintenance of adrenal cortex
   Promotes secretion of steroids, oxidative phosphorylation in adrenal cortex
   Mobilizes and increases oxidation of free fatty acids in adipose tissue
   Increases gluconeogenesis in liver; increases cyclic AMP in adrenal cortex
   Decreases urea formation in liver

9. **Deficiency Diseases, Disorders:** Adrenal insufficiency; hypopituitarism; Addison's disease (deficiency); Cushing's syndrome (excess); Simmonds' disease (deficiency)

10. **Essentiality for Life**
    One of the most essential hormones—absence causes notable shortening of normal life span

CHEMISTRY

1. **Structure**
   Straight chain, simple polypeptide, 39 amino acids, $C_{214}H_{386}O_{93}N_{56}S$. Structure known and synthesized. Human ACTH: Ser—Tyr—Ser—Met—Glu—His—Phe—Arg—Try—Gly—Lys—Pro—Val—Gly—Lys—Lys—Arg—Arg—Pro—Val—Lys—Val—Tyr—Pro—Asp—Ala—Gly—Glu—Asp—Glu—Ser—Ala—Glu—Ala—Phe—Pro—Leu—Glu—Phe
   No S—S bridges
   Amino acids #1-24 essential, same in all species

2. **Reactions**

Heat—Stable	Alkali
Acid	Inactivates
Weak—stable	Hydrolysis
Strong—hydrolysis	Water—Soluble, acidic

Oxidation
   Irreversibly inactivates using
      periodate
   Reversibly inactivates using H_2O_2
Reduction—Stable

Light—Stable
Proteolysis—50% digestion of
   C-terminal end leaves
   active core

3. Properties

Appearance—White powder
MW—4500 (39 amino acids)
MP—No data
Crystal Form—No data
Salts—No data
Important Groups for Activity
   Methionine—redox center—
   reacts with thiol; if change
   proline at #12, 19, 24 or
   serine #1, lose activity; 1-24
   essential

Solubility
   H_2O—Freely sol.
   Acet., Alc.—Sol. in 60% alc.,
      60% Acet.
   Benz., Chl., Eth.—Insol.
Absn. Max.—Approx. 280 mμ
Chemical Nature—Acidic
   polypeptide
Misc.—pI = 4.65-4.80

4. Commercial Production

Extract pig, cattle, sheep, whale pituitaries
Synthetic production possible

5. Isolation

Sources—Pituitaries of various animals
Method
   Extract with 1 N acetic acid; precipitate with ethanol
   Adsorb on and elute from oxycellulose; freeze-dry
   Countercurrent distribution—500X purification using s-butanol—0.2%
      TCA
   Zone electrophoresis, end group analysis, analytical ultracentrifuga-
      tion

6. Determination

Bioassay
   Maintenance of weight of adrenal gland in hypophysectomized rats
   Depletion of vit. C in adrenals of hypophysectomized rats
   Involution of thymus
Physicochemical
Immunoassay
Radioimmunoassay

MEDICAL AND BIOLOGICAL ROLE

1. Species Occurrence, Specificity, Antigenicity
   Occurrence—All vertebrates
   Specificity—Slight biological differences, species differences located in
       sequence of amino acids 25-34
   Antigenicity—Slight

2. **Units:**   1 USP unit = 1 I.U. = 1.14 mg

3. **Normal Blood Levels (Man):**   0.0005 unit/100 ml

4. Administration
   Injection—Intravenous, intramuscular, subcutaneous
   Topical—No data
   Oral—Active (stimulates release of cortisol)

5. Factors Affecting Release
   Inhibitors—Increased plasma level glucocorticoids (feedback)
   Stimulators
       Cortical release factors (CRH)—diurnal rhythm
       Vasopressin, increased hepatic inactivation
       Epinephrine, histamine
       Stimulation of median eminence
       Psychic trauma (via hypothalamus)
       Decreased level of glucocorticoids

6. Deficiency Symptoms
   Decreased weight of adrenal (atrophy)
   Decreased mobilization of free fatty acids
   Decreased steroids in blood, urine (17-hydroxy and 17-keto)
   Fasting hypoglycemia
   Increased insulin sensitivity

7. Effects of Overdose, Excess
   Increased cortical secretions → hypertrophy → destruction
   Increased pigmentation
   Death
   Hypersensitivity

METABOLIC ROLE

1. **Biosynthesis**
   Precursors—16 of 20 standard amino acids. No Cys, Thr, Ile or Asn
   Intermediates—MSH (?)

2. **Production Sites:** Anterior pituitary—basophilic cells; placenta

3. **Storage Areas:** Anterior pituitary

4. **Blood Carriers:** Free and combined with plasma proteins

5. **Half-life:** 15 min

6. **Target Tissues:** Adrenal cortex, perirenal cells, embryonic rest cells

7. **Reactions**
   Reactive intermediate: cyclic AMP—Secondary messenger

Organ	Enzyme System	Effect
Adrenal cortex	Adenyl cyclase	Activated
	Phosphorylase b	Activated
	Cholesterol 20-Hydroxylase	Activated

8. **Mode of Action**
   Cellular—
   Anabolic—
   Increases melanin synthesis in skin
   Increases steroid synthesis in adrenal
   Increases protein synthesis in liver (via cortisol)
   Catabolic
   Increases glycogenolysis (adrenal cortex)
   Increases gluconeogenesis (liver) (via cortisol)
   Increases lipolysis and oxidation of fatty acids in adipose tissue
   Other:
   Increases oxidative phosphorylation in adrenal cortex
   Increases production of cyclic AMP to produce $NADPH_2$ in adrenal
   cortex
   Decreases cholesterol in adrenal cortex
   Organismal
   Increases weight of adrenals, depletes cortex of vit. C.
   Mobilizes free fatty acids from adipose tissue

Hypoglycemic, reduces urea formation
Increases iodine uptake by thyroid
Stimulates secretion of gluco- and mineralocorticoids by adrenal cortex
Stimulates melanophores, darkening of skin

9. Catabolism
Intermediates—Liver destruction
Excretion Products—Free in urine (very little)

MISCELLANEOUS

1. Relationship to Vitamins
Vitamin C—Depleted in adrenal cortex on stimulation by ACTH
Niacin—Production of $NADPH_2$ by ACTH via cyclic AMP
Vitamin D—Antagonized indirectly by ACTH via cortisol action
Biotin and Vitamin A—Adrenocortical insufficiency noted in biotin and
vitamin A deficiency
Pantothenic acid, niacin—Synergistic with ACTH in steroid hormone
synthesis

2. Relationship to Other Hormones
Epinephrine—Synergist, stimulates release of ACTH.
Cortisol, corticosterone—Synergists or antagonists depending on concen-
tration. Production stimulated by ACTH
CRH—Stimulates release of ACTH
Vasopressin—Similar to CRH, in action
T4 and TSH—ACTH stimulates iodine uptake by thyroid
MSH—MSH is a part of ACTH molecule
Insulin—Antagonist to ACTH
STH—Antagonist (protein metab.) synergist (fat metab.)

3. Unusual Features
Reversible loss of activity on oxidation with H_2O_2
Reacts with thiols
Irreversible deactivation by periodate
First 13 amino acids essential for corticotropic activity
Full activity at first 20 amino acids
MSH, a part of ACTH, and its activity increased by N-acetylation
Second messenger (cyclic AMP) involved in adrenal cortex

4. **Possible Relationships of Deficiency to Metabolic Action**
> Atrophy of adrenal cortex—Lack of stimulus from ACTH
>
> Decreased mobilization of fatty acids—Decreased glucocorticoids, increased insulin activity
>
> Decreased steroids in blood and urine—Decreased production of adrenal corticoids
>
> Fasting hypoglycemia—Decreased gluconeogenesis
>
> Increased insulin sensitivity—Insulin antagonism to ACTH and cortisol

23
Melanocyte-Stimulating Hormone (MSH)

GENERAL INFORMATION

1. **Synonyms:** Melanophore (affecting) hormone, melanophore-stimulating hormone, melanotrophin, melanotrophic hormone, chromatophorotropic hormone, melanosome-dispersing hormone, pigmentation hormone, β-hormone

2. **History**
   - 1932—Zondek and Krohn noted factor in intermediate lobe mediating pigmentary responses in lower vertebrates
   - 1954—Lerner proposed term melanocyte-stimulating hormone for above factor
   - 1956—Geschwind *et al.* isolated β-MSH from pig pituitary
   - 1957—Harris and Lerner isolated α-MSH from pig pituitary tissue
   - 1959—Harris and Roos isolated β-MSH from bovine pituitary
   - 1960—Dixon isolated β-MSH from human pituitary
   - 1960—Hofmann *et al.* synthesized derivatives of β-MSH
   - 1960—Li, Dixon isolated α-MSH from horse pituitary
   - 1960—Lee *et al.* determined structure of α-MSH
   - 1963—Schwyzer *et al.* synthesized α-MSH and β-MSH

3. **Physiological Forms**
   l-α-MSH, l-β-MSH (intermedin) (approx equal biological activity)

4. **Active Analogs and Related Compounds**
    Acetylated N-terminal (β-MSH and ACTH)
    Common heptapeptide (Met–Glu–His–Phe–Arg–Try–Gly) of α,β-MSH
    and ACTH

5. **Inactive Analogs and Related Compounds**
    ACTH (1% of MSH activity)
    Hydrolyzed fragments of MSH

6. **Antagonists:**   Cortisone, d-amino acid analogs (competitive inhibitors),
    melatonin

7. **Synergists:**   STH, TSH (amphibia), caffeine, theophylline

8. **Physiological Functions**
    Function in mammals is obscure (protection from sunlight?), small effect
    on skin pigmentation
    Expands or contracts pigments in various chromatophores
    Expands melanophore pigments with color changes in amphibia (adapta-
    tion to environment); weak ACTH activity; adipokinetic effect,
    stimulates T4 secretion
    Increases sensitivity to light, decreases dark adaptation time (lower
    vertebrates)

9. **Deficiency Diseases, Disorders**
    Excess—Addison's disease, adrenal insufficiency (darkening)
    Deficiency—Hypopituitarism (light)

10. **Essentiality for Life:**   Not required; present in all vertebrates with
    differing functions

CHEMISTRY

1. **Structure**
    Polypeptide—purified, synthesized, α and β-forms, straight chains
    α, 13 amino acids—Ser–Tyr–Ser–[Met–Glu–His–Phe–Arg–Try–
    Gly]–Lys–Pro–Val
    N-terminal = CH_3CO-, C-terminal = $-NH_2$ similar all species
    β18 amino acids in all species except 22 in human—Ala–Glu–Lys–
    Lys–Asp–Glu–Gly–Pro–Tyr–Arg–Met–Glu–His–Phe–Arg–
    Try–Gly–Ser–Pro–Pro–Lys–Asp
    No S–S bridges

2. Reactions

Heat—Stable
Acid—Stable
Alkali—Stable (potentiates)
Water—Sol., basic

Oxidation—H_2O_2 reversibly inactivates
Reduction—thiols reversibly inactivate
Light—No effect
Proteolysis—Decreases activity

3. Properties

Appearance—White powder
MW—α 1500 (13 A.A.)
β 2100-2600 (18-22 A.A.)
Crystal Form—No data
Salts—No data
Important Groups for Activity
Met (redox center)
Tyr
Common hepapeptide in all α's, β's, and ACTH
(Met———Gly)

Solubility
H_2O—Sol.
Acet., Alc.—Insol.
Benz., Chl., Eth.—Insol.
Absn. Max.—Approx. 280 mμ
Chemical Nature
Simple, peptides (α—acidic, β—basic)
α-MSH: $\alpha_D^{25} = 58.5°C$ (10% acetic acid)
Misc—pI = α 5.5-7.0, β 11.0

4. **Commercial Production:**   Synthetic

5. Isolation

Sources—Human, pig, bovine, pituitary glands, urine, blood
Methods
β-MSH
Extract with KCl at pH 5.5; precipitate with salt; adsorb on oxycellulose
Purify via carboxylic acid resin
Countercurrent distribution (1.2 M urea, 0.2 M ethylenediamine, 0.1 N HCl)

6. Determination

Bioassay—Darkening of frog skin ($\alpha > \beta$)
Physicochemical
Photoelectric reflectance assay
Immunoasay
Radioimmunoassay

MEDICAL AND BIOLOGICAL ROLE

1. **Species Occurrence, Specificity, and Antigenicity**
   Occurrence: All vertebrates (α-MSH, β-MSH). All preparations similar in
   activity from all animals
   Specificity
   α-MSH—Slight species differences in activity
   β-MSH—Definite species differences in activity
   Antigenicity: α—None. β—Slight

2. **Units:**   Relative to posterior pituitary standard or by weight

3. **Normal Blood Levels (Man):**   0.09 mμg/ml or less

4. **Administration**
   Injection—Subcutaneous
   Topical—Active, used in amphibian experiments
   Oral—Active, used in amphibian experiments

5. **Factors Affecting Release**
   Inhibitors—MIF via hypothalamus, epinephrine, nervous controls, mela-
   tonin
   Stimulators—Metabolic, nervous controls, MRH via hypothalamus

6. **Deficiency Symptoms**
   Lightened skin color (amphibians)
   Chromatophore contraction
   Guanophore expansion

7. **Effects of Overdose, Excess**
   Darkening of skin (amphibians and humans), temporary
   Hyperglycemia

METABOLIC ROLE

1. **Biosynthesis**
   Precursors—13-14 of 20 standard amino acids. Missing (Cys, Asn, Gln,
   Leu, Ile, Thr, Val)
   Intermediates—Unknown

2. **Production Sites**
   Intermediate lobe of pituitary, except in birds, whales, elephants,
   armadillos, where it is in anterior lobe
   Also in posterior lobes

3. **Storage Areas:**   In intermediate lobe of pituitary

4. **Blood Carriers:**   Free and combined with plasma proteins

5. **Half-life:**   1—2 hrs.

6. **Target Tissues:**   Skin (melanophores) (amphibia)

7. **Reactions**
   Reactive intermediates: Cyclic AMP (secondary messenger)

Organ	Enzyme System	Effect
Skin	Adenyl cyclase	Activated
	Tyrosinase, see ACTH enzymes	Activated

8. **Mode of Action**
   Cellular
   　Anabolic—Melanin formation
   　Catabolic—Blocks glycolytic pathways
   　Other—Increases permeability to Na^+, changes protoplasmic viscosity.
   　　Expands pigments in melanophores
   Organismal
   　ACTH function (weak)
   　Blocks action of melatonin
   　Regulates skin color changes, light adaptations

9. **Catabolism**
   Intermediates—Unknown
   Excretion products—Free in urine; also breakdown products

MISCELLANEOUS

1. **Relationship to Vitamins**
   Vitamin C—Adrenal cortex depleted on ACTH and MSH activity
   Vitamin A—MSH decreases dark adaptation time

2. **Relationship to Other Hormones**
   STH, TSH—Synergists to MSH
   T4—Secretion stimulated by MSH
   Cortisone, melatonin—Antagonist to MSH
   Epinephrine—Inhibitor of MSH release

3. Unusual Features

Very resistant to degradation or inactivation
Reversibly inactivated by oxidation (H_2O_2)
Reduced with thiols
Heptapeptide 4-10 similar to ACTH
α and β forms with similar activity but different a.a. contents

4. Possible Relationships of Deficiency to Metabolic Action

Lightened skin color (amphibia)—No MSH available to promote melanin
dispersion

24
Oxytocin

GENERAL INFORMATION

1. Synonyms: Oxytocic hormone, postlobin-O, posterior-lobe principle, Pitocin, lactogogin, uteracon, α-hypophamine

2. History

1906—Dale noted effect of posterior pituitary factor in stimulating uterine contraction

1928—Kamin *et al.* separated two active fractions from neural lobe: one was active in raising blood pressure in mammals; the other promoted uterine contractions

1952—Pierce *et al.* isolated oxytocin

1953—du Vigneaud *et al.* synthesized oxytocin

1965—Flouret *et al.* synthesized d-oxytocin

3. Physiological Forms: l-oxytocin

4. Active Analogs and Related Compounds

Vasopressin

Isotocin (some fishes)

8-Isoleucine oxytocin (other fishes, amphibia)

Arginine vasotocin (all vertebrates, except mammals)

5. Inactive Analogs and Related Compounds

Reduced form of oxytocin, enlarged or smaller ring forms, forms with side chains removed

6. **Antagonists:**   2'-o-methyltyrosine oxytocin

7. **Synergists**
   Uterus—Prolactin, relaxin, estradiol
   Mammary gland—STH, progesterone, estradiol, T4, cortisol

8. **Physiological Functions**
   Uterine contraction, milk ejection, facilitates sperm ascent in female
   tract
   Decreases: Membrane potential of myometrium; BMR, liver glycogen
   Stimulates oviposition in hen, releases LH
   Increases: Blood sugar, urinary Na and K

9. **Deficiency Diseases, Disorders**
   Insufficiency of labor, atonic uterine bleeding

10. **Essentiality for Life:**   Not essential

CHEMISTRY

1. **Structure:**
   Octapeptide—synthesized
   Cys—Tyr—Ile—Gln—Asn—Cys—Pro—Leu—Gly—(NH$_2$)
   Oxytocin—$C_{43}H_{66}N_{12}O_{12}S_2$

2. **Reactions**

Heat—No data	Oxidation—Stable
Acid—Stable, (weak), unstable (strong)	Reduction—Inactivates (ring opens)
	Light—No data
Alkali—Unstable	Proteolysis by chymotripsin,
Water—Sol., basic	trypsin or tyrosinase inactivates

3. **Properties**

Appearance—Amorphous white powder	Solubility
	H$_2$O—Soluble
MW—1007	Acet., Alc.—Sl. Sol., Sol.
MP—No data	Benz., Chl., Ether—Insol.
Crystal Form—No data	Absn. Max.—Approx. 280 mμ
Salts—Citrate, flavianate	Chemical Nature—Basic octapeptide
Important Groups for Activity	$\alpha_D^{22} = -26.2°$
Ile, Glu, Asp, Leu, Gly, Cys	Misc.—pI = 7.7
Ring (opening inactivates)	

4. **Commercial Production**
>Synthetic, from amino acids
>Posterior pituitary lobe of cattle, sheep (extraction)

5. **Isolation**
>Sources—Posterior lobe of pituitary, cattle
>Methods
>>Dissociate from protein with acid hydrolysis
>>Electrodialysis, precipitation
>>DEAE cellulose, pH 5.5

6. **Determination**
>Bioassay
>>Blood pressure drop in chick
>>Milk ejection in rat
>>Contraction of isolated, uterus of virgin guinea pig
>Physicochemical—No information

MEDICAL AND BIOLOGICAL ROLE

1. **Species Occurrence, Specificity, and Antigenicity**
>Occurrence: Found in most vertebrates, in slightly different forms
>Specificity: Interspecies reactivity—Decrease in action in lower forms
>Antigenicity: Low

2. **Units:**   1 USP unit = approx. 2 μg of pure hormone

3. **Normal Blood Levels (Man):**   0.15-1.5 milliunits/100 ml plasma

4. **Administration**
>Injection—intramuscular, subcutaneous, I.V. drip
>Topical—Nasal spray
>Oral—Inactivated by chymotrypsin in intestine

5. **Factors Affecting Release**
>Inhibitors: No data
>Stimulants: Reflex arcs—Chemical and neural reflexes from suckling, milking, from cervix, vagina (dilatation of birth canal); psychic events; relaxin

6. **Deficiency Symptoms**
    Delayed uterine contraction in pregnancy
    Decreased milk flow

7. **Effects of Overdose, Excess**
    Tetanic contraction of pregnant uterus
    Increase in milk flow

METABOLIC ROLE

1. **Biosynthesis**
    Precursors—8 of 20 std amino acids. Missing are Glu, Asp, Met, Arg, Lys,
        His, Pro, Try, Phe, Ala, Thr, Ser
    Intermediates: Neurophysin—Peptide complex

2. **Production Sites:**   Hypothalamus (paraventricular nuclei?)

3. **Storage Areas:**   Posterior pituitary and hypothalamus

4. **Blood Carriers:**   Unbound and in loose association with plasma proteins

5. **Half-life:**   9 min in pregnant woman

6. **Target Tissues:**   Uterus (pregnant), mammary gland, other smooth muscle

7. **Reactions:**   Reactive form—No data

8. **Mode of Action**
    Cellular
        Anabolic—No data
        Catabolic—No data
        Other—Contraction of myoepithelial cells around mammary alveoli.
            Contraction of uterine smooth muscle
    Organismal
        Uterine contraction
        Milk ejection
        Vasodilator ⎫
        Antidiuretic ⎭ in large doses only

9. Catabolism
    Intermediates
        In pregnancy, plasma oxytocinase inactivates
        Oxytocinase formed in placenta breaks down oxytocin
        Removed from plasma by liver, *kidney*, and mammary gland
    Excretion products: A little, free in urine

MISCELLANEOUS

1. Relationship to Vitamins: No data

2. Relationship to Hormones
    Vasopressin
        Structurally similar to vasopressin
        Always secreted with vasopressin irrespective of stimulus
    Prolactin—Oxytocin may stimulate release of prolactin
    STH, TSH, ACTH, LH, FSH, Prol.—Anterior pituitary hormones; related
        in milk production
    Estradiol—Uterine effect dependent on estrogen presence.
    LH—oxytocin stimulates LH release
    Norepinephrine ⎫
    Serotonin   ⎬ Occur with oxytocin in posterior pituitary
    CRH—Structural similarity to oxytocin
    Relaxin—Stimulates oxytocin release

3. Unusual Features
    Very similar structurally to vasopressin but main physiological actions
        very different (only two amino acids differ)
    No known function in male mammal
    Protein, neurophysin, binds neurohypophysial hormones specifically
    Always secreted with vasopressin irrespective of nature of stimulus
    Nonpregnant uterus is more sensitive to ADH than to oxytocin
    Vasodilator effect of oxytocin is blocked by ADH
    Releases anterior pituitary hormones in fish
    Increases oviposition in birds and reptiles
    Increases spawning reflex in fish

4. Possible Relationships of Deficiency Symptoms to Metabolic Action: No
        data

25
Vasopressin

GENERAL INFORMATION

1. **Synonyms:** Arginine vasopressin, ADH (antidiuretic hormone) anti-
   diuretin, Pitressin, β-hypophamine, Tonephin, Vasophysin

2. **History**
   - 1895—Oliver and Schafer noted effect of posterior pituitary factor on
     rise in blood pressure
   - 1937—Gilman and Goodman showed dehydration increased plasma and
     urine levels of vasopressin
   - 1942—Van Dyke isolated crude protein fraction possessing oxytocin and
     vasopressin activities from oxen pituitaries
   - 1953-54—DuVigneaud *et al.* determined structure and synthesized ADH

3. **Physiological Forms:** l-vasopressin

4. **Active Analogs and Related Compounds**
   Arginine vasopressin (most mammals)
   Lysine vasopressin (pig)
   Vasotocin (birds, amphibia, fish)

5. **Inactive Analogs and Related Compounds**
   Opening of ring; removal of side chain
   Change in size of ring

6. **Antagonists:** Norepinephrine, certain prostaglandins

7. **Synergists:**   Aldosterone, STH, prolactin, corticosterone, T4, testosterone, epinephrine

8. **Physiological Functions**
    Elevates blood pressure (mammals) (reverse effect in birds)
    Decreases kidney blood flow
    Antidiuretic, acts as CRF, releases ACTH
    Increases NaCl and urea excretion
    Regulates water balance
    Stimulates contraction of smooth muscles
    Increases renal tubular H_2O reabsorption
    Releases anterior pituitary hormones

9. **Deficiency Diseases, Disorders**
    Deficiency—Diabetes insipidus
    Excess—Schwartz-Bartter syndrome (oat-cell carcinoma)

10. **Essentiality for Life:**   Not essential

CHEMISTRY

1. **Structure**
    Octapeptide—synthesized
    Cys—Tyr—Phe—Gln—Asn—Cys—Pro—Arg—Gly(NH_2)
    Arginine vasopressin, $C_{46}H_{65}N_{15}O_{12}S_2$

2. **Reactions**

    Heat—Degrades in solution
    Acid—Stable
    Alkali—Unstable
    Water—Soluble, basic

    Oxidation—Stable
    Reduction—Inactivates (ring opens)
    Light—Unstable
    Proteolysis inactivates (by trypsin (which removes terminal glycine amide group), but not by pepsin)

3. **Properties**

    Appearance—amorphous
      white powder
    MW—1084 (arginine-vasopressin)
    MP—No data
    Crystal Form—No data
    Salts, Esters—Tannate

    Important Groups for Activity
      Cyclic pentapeptide (opening inactivates)
      Tripeptide side chain
      Cys

Solubility
  H_2O—Soluble
  Alc.—Sol.
  Acet., Benz., Chl., Eth.—Insol.

Absn. Max.—Approx. 280 mμ
Chemical Nature—Basic peptide
Misc.—pI = 10.9

4. Commercial Production

Synthesized from amino acids.
Posterior lobe of pituitary of domestic animals (hog, beef)

5. Isolation

Sources: Posterior pituitary glands (hog, beef)
Methods:
  Acetic acid extraction of posterior pituitary powder
  Percolation through Celite using 70% ethanol and gradually increasing
    concentrations of water and acetic acid
  Or the neurophysin peptide complex is extracted with acetic acid and
    the protein precipitated with NaCl. Treatment with trichloroacetic
    acid then dissociates the complex and precipitates the protein

6. Determination

Bioassay
  Blood pressure measurements on cats, dogs, or chickens
  Diuretic studies on dogs, rats, and rabbits
  Weight gain in frogs
Physiochemical: Radioimmunoassay

MEDICAL AND BIOLOGICAL ROLE

1. Species Occurrence, Specificity, and Antigenicity

Occurrence
  Vasopressin-like substances found in vertebrates from cyclostomes
    through mammals
  Loss of activity as go to amphibia and fish
Specificity—Decreasing interspecies reactivity in lower vertebrates
Antigenicity—Low

2. Units: 1 USP posterior pituitary unit = 1 international posterior pituitary
unit = 0.5 mg of the international standard oxytocic, vasopressor,
and antidiuretic substances (ox posterior pituitary)

3. Normal Blood Levels (Man):   3.7 milliunits/100 ml

4. **Administration**
   Injection—Intravenous, intramuscular, or subcutaneous
   Topical—Inhalation of powders or sprays
   Oral—No data

5. **Factors Affecting Release**
   Inhibitors
      Low osmotic pressure in blood
      Ethyl alcohol
      High extracellular fluid volume
   Stimulators
      High blood osmotic pressure
      Acetylcholine, lobeline
      Physostigmine
      Cold, low fluid volume
      Hemorrhage
      Morphine, nicotine, ether, some barbiturates, tranquilizers, and general anesthetics
      Ca^{++}-ion-(inhibits binding to protein)
      Stress
      Exercise, psychic events

6. **Deficiency Symptoms**
   Diuresis
   Polydipsia
   Decreased NaCl and urea excretion

7. **Effects of Overdose, Excess**
   Increased water reabsorption, blood pressure
   Smooth muscle contraction—G.I. activity
   Facial pallor
   Uterine cramps
   Coronary circulation complications

METABOLIC ROLE

1. **Biosynthesis**
   Precursors—Eight of standard 20 amino acids. Missing are Glu, Asp, Met, Lys, His, Leu, Prol, Try, Ile, Ala, Thre, Ser
   Intermediates—Neurophysin-peptide complex

2. **Production Sites:**   Hypothalamus, esp. supraoptic nuclei. Secreted into neurohypophysis

3. **Storage Areas:**   Hypothalamus and posterior pituitary

4. **Blood Carriers:**   Unbound, and loose association with plasma protein

5. **Half-life:**   In plasma, 8 min

6. **Target Tissues:**   Capillaries, arterioles, coronary vessels, kidney tubules, smooth muscle

7. **Reactions**

    Reactive intermediate: Cyclic AMP—secondary messenger

Organ	Enzyme System	Effect
Kidney	Hyaluronidase	Activated
Kidney (distal tubule)	Adenyl cyclase	Activated

8. **Mode of Action**

    Cellular

    Anabolic—No data

    Catabolic—Depolymerizes hyaluronic acid

    Other

    Increases passive permeability of epithelium of distal segment of nephron to water; allows osmotic forces to operate more freely

    Increases intracellular water in muscle; decreases Na and K

    Increases pore size or number in cell membrane

    Organismal

    Antidiuretic

    Decreases coronary blood flow

    Increases motility of bowel

    Arterial smooth muscle sensitized to effects of norepinephrine by physiological amounts of ADH

    Renal blood flow reduced by ADH

9. **Catabolism**

    Intermediates—Inactivated in kidney and liver

    Excretion Products: Some free in urine

MISCELLANEOUS

1. **Relationship to Vitamins:**   No data

2. **Relationship to Other Hormones**

   Oxytocin, Hypertensin—Structurally very similar to vasopressin but main physiological effect is very different

   Aldosterone, Corticosterone—Synergistic with vasopressin; related to antidiuretic activity of vasopressin

   CRF—Vasopressin suggested to have CRF (corticotropin release factor) properties

   STH, T4, Testosterone, Prolactin—Synergistic with vasopressin

   Aldosterone—ADH and aldosterone may interact in water and electrolyte conservation

   Norepinephrine, Prostaglandins—Norepinephrine and certain prostaglandins inhibit ADH activity in kidney

3. **Unusual Features**

   Thiazides which act as diuretics, paradoxically reduce polyuria in both pituitary diabetes insipidus and nephrogenic diabetes insipidus. May act by reducing filtration rate

   Nonpregnant uterus is more sensitive to ADH than to oxytocin. Rare form of diabetes insipidus is not caused by lack of ADH but by inability of kidney tubule to respond to ADH. (An inborn error of metabolism)

   Reverse effects in birds

   Increases skin permeability in amphibia

4. **Possible Relationships of Deficiency Symptoms to Metabolic Action**

   Decreased NaCl and urea excretion—Permeability of epithelium of distal segment of nephron to water is reduced and water reabsorption is decreased

26
Thyroxine

GENERAL INFORMATION

1. **Synonyms:** T_4, 3,5,3',5'-tetraiodothyronine

2. **History**

16th Century—Anon. Cretinism described
1825—Parry associated enlarged thyroid with exophthalmia, tachycardia
1874—Gull associated atrophy of thyroid with characteristic syndrome
1891—Murray treated hypothyroidism with injection of thyroid extract
1896—Baumann showed that thyroid contains iodine
1911—Baumann demonstrated diiodotyrosine in thyroid
1915—Kendall isolated and crystallized thyroxine
1926—Harington determined structural formula
1927—Harington and Barger synthesized thyroxine
1951—Gross *et al.* isolated and identified triiodothyronine as active factor in thyroid

3. **Physiological Forms:** l-thyroxine, 3',3,5-triiodothyronine (T_3, TRIT), tetraiodothyroacetic acid (TETRAC), triiodothyroacetic acid (TRIAC)

4. **Active Analogs and Related Compounds**

d-thyroxine (fractional activity of l-thyroxine)
Triiodothyropropionic acid (very active in tadpole metamorphosis)

5. **Inactive Analogs and Related Compounds:** Deiodinated T4; T4 with esterified hydroxyl group

6. **Antagonists:** 3,3',5'-triiodothyronine, guanethidine; 2',6'-diiodotyrosine, insulin, PTH

7. **Synergists:** STH, cortisol, epinephrine, prolactin, MSH, oxytocin, progesterone, vasopressin

8. **Physiological Functions**
   Regulates growth, differentiation, oxidative metabolism, electrolytic balance
   Increases CHO metabolism, calorigenesis, protein anabolism, BMR, O_2 consumption, fat catabolism, fertility
   Sensitizes nervous system

9. **Deficiency Diseases, Disorders**
   Deficiency—Cretinism, goiter (deficient), Hashimoto's disease, Gull's disease, myxedema
   Excess—Grave's disease, thyrotoxicosis, thyroiditis, goiter

10. **Essentiality for Life**
    Required for development and growth of all vertebrates
    Deficiency in adult shortens life span

CHEMISTRY

1. **Structure:**

Thyroxine, $C_{15}H_{11}I_4NO_4$

2. **Reactions**

Heat—Decomposes at $231°C$	Oxidation—Unstable
Acid—Unstable (Sol. in acid alc.)	Reduction—Stable
	Light—Unstable
Alkali—Sol. in alk. alc.	Enzyme action: Unstable to
Water—Insol.	deiodinating enzymes.

3. **Properties**

   Appearance—White crystalline
      powder
   MW—776.9
   MP—231-233°C decomp.
   Crystal Form—needle-like
   Salts—Sodium
   Important Groups for Activity
      —l-Alanine
      —O—
      —I (all 4 positions)
      —OH

   Solubility
      H_2O—Insol.
      Acet.—Insol.
      Alc.—Sol. at acid or alk. pH
      Benz., Chl., Eth.—Insol.
   Absn. Max.—231 mμ
   Chemical Nature
      Acidic substituted amino acid
   α_D = —4.4° (aq. alk. EtOH)
   Misc.—pK_a = 2.2, (COOH), 6.45 (OH),
      10.1 (NH_2)
      pI = 3.5

4. **Commercial Production**

   Synthetic and from pig thyroid by defatting and drying with acetone—
      thyroid, U.S.P.
   Sodium salts
      Sodium levothyroxine, USP (synthroid)
      Sodium liothyronine, USP (cytomel)

5. **Isolation**

   Sources—Pig thyroid
   Method—Extraction:
      Proteolysis, pH 8.4, (pancreatin and trypsin) of thyroid, 24 hr at 37°C
      Extract with n-butanol saturated with N HCl
      Paper chromatography or ion-exchange resin
      Partition chromatography (kieselguhr in 0.5 N NaOH) separates T_4
         from T_3

6. **Determination**

   Bioassay
      Metamorphosis in tadpoles
      Increased oxidative metabolism
   Physicochemical—Protein-bound iodine (PBI) in plasma. Radioassay

MEDICAL AND BIOLOGICAL ROLE

1. **Species Occurrence, Specificity, and Antigenicity**
   Occurrence
       All vertebrates have thyroid tissue, but follicles dispersed in lampreys
           and bony fish
       Thyroxine and precursors found in various invertebrates but no
           follicles
   Specificity
       Interreactive all vertebrates; no loss in potency (i.e. no specificity)
       No response in invertebrates; different functions in lower vertebrates
   Antigenicity—No antigenicity

2. **Units:**   In mg

3. **Normal Blood Levels (Man):**   3.0-6.5 μg/100 ml serum

4. **Administration:**
       Injection—No data
       Topical—No data
       Oral—Thyroid tablets, sodium levothyroxine, sodium liothyroxine

5. **Factors Affecting Release**
   Inhibitors
       High blood I_2
       High blood T_4—feedback via hypothalamus
       Stress, pain
   Stimulators
       TSH
       Low blood T_4—feedback via hypothalamus
       Cold
       Direct nervous control

6. **Deficiency Symptoms (Humans)**
       Tumors of pituitary
       Decreased BMR
       Accumulation of mucoprotein
       Increase in blood lipid and cholesterol
       Increase in liver gluconeogenesis
       Extracellular retention of NaCl and H_2O

7. **Effects of Overdose, Excess**
   Acceleration of growth, maturation
   Increased BMR, esp. liver, skin, kidney, smooth muscle, gastric mucosa
   Decreased tissue glycogen
   Increased blood sugar
   Exophthalmos
   Hyperthyroidism, Graves's disease
   Thyrotoxicosis

METABOLIC ROLE

1. **Biosynthesis:** Tyrosine → Monoiodotyrosine → Diiodotyrosine → Thyroxine Site(s) in Cell—Data not conclusive

2. **Production Sites:** Thyroid gland

3. **Storage Areas:** Colloid in thyroid follicles = thyroglobulin

4. **Blood Carriers**
   α-Globulin
   Acid glycoprotein
   Albumin

5. **Half-life:** 6-7 days

6. **Target Tissues:** Systemic—All tissues, esp. adenohypophysis, hypothalamus

7. **Reactions**
   Reactive intermediate: Cyclic AMP—secondary messenger

Organ	Enzyme System	Effect
	67 tissue enzymes affected *in vivo*	
Thyroid	Mitochondrial enzyme systems	Activated
Thyroid	TCA cycle—oxidative phosphorylating enzymes	Uncoupled
Thyroid	Adenyl cyclase	Activated

8. **Mode of Action**
   Cellular
   Anabolic
   Increases protein synthesis on the ribosomes and $_m$RNA synthesis in muscle, kidney, reticulocytes, liver

Catabolic

Increases protein catabolism in brain, spleen, and testis

Increases glucose and fat catabolism

Other—Swells mitochondria, affects permeability, regulates redox potential, chelates metals that inhibit enzymes

Uncouples mitochondrial oxidative phosphorylation at 2 points

Decreases mucoprotein synthesis

Organismal

Stimulates hematopoiesis, oögenesis, spermatogenesis, lactation, intestinal absorption

Regulates growth, differentiation, electrolyte balance, heat production, O_2 consumption, BMR

Sensitizes nervous system

9. **Catabolism**

Intermediates

Iodine split off in liver, kidney, salivary glands, and recycled

Residue coupled with glucuronic acid or sulfate and excreted. Also oxidative deamination of amino acid residues

Excretion Products

Compounds containing diphenyl ether and at least two carbons of side chain excreted as glucuronides and sulfates in bile

Very small amounts free in urine and bile

MISCELLANEOUS

1. **Relationship to Vitamins**

Vitamin A—T_4 needed for vit. A synthesis in liver

B—Complex vitamin deficiencies develop in hyperthyroidism

Vit B_{12}—T4 aids in B_{12} absorption

Vitamin C—Synergist in cold survival

Niacin—Synergist in mitochondrial metabolism

2. **Relationship to Other Hormones**

STH, ACTH, FSH, LH, TSH, Prolactin—synergists to T4 esp. in lactation

ACTH—Antagonist in proper relative concentration

Insulin—T4 stimulates secretion of insulin

TSH—Stimulates production of T4

FSH—Inhibited by T4

MSH, ACTH—Stimulate iodine uptake by thyroid

PTH—Antagonist to T4
Cortisol—Synergist to T4

3. Unusual Features

Powerful chelating agent, esp. with Mg
Free OH participates in quinonoid formation
Regulates metamorphosis in amphibia
Osmoregulatory in fish
Iodinated tyrosine found in invertebrate exoskeleton—inactive
Diffuse thyroid gland in teleosts & other lower forms
TRIAC—potent stimulant for metamorphosis
TETRAC—potent metabolic stimulant
Decreased activity if I is replaced with Br or Cl
Decreased activity if OH is removed or I position changed

4. Possible Relationships of Deficiency Symptoms to Metabolic Action

Decreased BMR—Lack of T_4 stimulus for anabolism
Accumulation of Mucoprotein—Lack of T_4 control of mucoprotein
   synthesis
Increase in Blood Lipid and Cholesterol—Decreased fat catabolism
Increase in Liver Gluconeogenesis—Antagonism by ACTH (cortisol)
Extracellular Retention of NaCl and H_2O—Antagonism by ACTH and
   aldosterone (?)

27
Parathyroid
Hormone

GENERAL INFORMATION

1. **Synonyms:** PTH, Parathormone

2. **History**
   - 1900—Vassale and Generali reported convulsions and tetany from removal of parathyroids only
   - 1909—MacCallum and Voegtlin reported effect of parathyroidectomy on plasma Ca
   - 1924-25—Hanson, Collip prepared active extracts from parathyroid gland
   - 1942—Patt and Luckhardt demonstrated that blood Ca level controls parathyroid secretion
   - 1959—Rasmussen, Aurbach prepared pure parathyroid hormone peptides

3. **Physiological Forms:** *l*-Parathormone

4. **Active Analogs and Related Compounds:** No data

5. **Inactive Analogs and Related Compounds:** No data

6. **Antagonists:** T4, STH, estradiol, testosterone, TCT

7. **Synergists:** Vitamin D, estrogens (birds), cortisol

8. **Physiological Functions**

Increases blood Ca, kidney Ca reabsorption, PO_4 excretion, blood citrate

Mobilizes Ca and PO_4 from bone.

Activates Ca and PO_4 absorption from G.I. tract (requires vitamin D)

Increases osteoclast formation

9. **Deficiency Diseases, Disorders**

Deficiency—Tetany, hypoparathyroidism

Excess—von Recklinghausen's disease, hyperparathyroidism

10. **Essentiality for Life:**   One of the most essential hormones. Absence rapidly leads to tetany and death of adult

CHEMISTRY

1. **Structure**

Simple polypeptide (83 amino acids), sequence determined

Straight chain—No S—S bridges

Ala———Leu

2. **Reactions**

Heat—No data

Acid—Stable, dilute, acid

Alkali—Relatively unstable

Water—Sol., acidic

Oxidation—H_2O_2, performic acid inactivate

Reduction—Stable

Light—No data

Proteolysis—Loses activity

3. **Properties**

Appearance—No data

MW—8500

MP—No data

Crystal Form—No data

Salts—No data

Important Groups for Activity

Met, Try, Tyr

Solubility

H_2O—Sol.

Acet., Alc.—Insol.

Benz., Chl., Eth.—Insol.

Absn. Max.—Approx. 280 mμ

Chemical Nature—Acidic polypeptide

Misc—pI = 4.8

4. **Commercial Production:**   From bovine parathyroid

5. **Isolation**

Sources—Bovine parathyroid

Methods
    Extraction
        Extract with 80% acetic acid
        Precipitate in 86% acetone
        Ultrafilter at pH 2.4
    Purification
        Column chromatography on Dowex 50
        Countercurrent distribution
        Gel filtration

6. Determination
    Bioassay
        Serum Ca increase in dogs
        Increase in urine P output
    Physicochemical
        Radioimmunoassay

MEDICAL AND BIOLOGICAL ROLE

1. Species Occurrence, Specificity, and Antigenicity
    Occurrence—Found in all vertebrates above fish and cyclostomes
    Specificity—Interspecific potency high, e.g. bovine and human Para-
        thormone—Isoactive
    Antigenicity—Low

2. Units: 1 USP unit = 1/100 the amount of PTH to increase dog blood Ca
    1 mg/100 ml in 18 hr after subcutaneous injection

3. Normal Blood Levels (Man): Est. 4000 USP units/100 ml plasma

4. Administration
    Injection—Parathyroid USP (Paroidin) usually subcutaneous; occasion-
        ally I.V.
    Topical—No data
    Oral—Destroyed by proteolytic enzymes

5. Factors Affecting Release
    Inhibitors—High serum Ca; vasomotor nerve control
    Stimulators—Low serum Ca feedback; vasomotor nerve control

6. **Deficiency Symptoms**
   Decreased blood (Ca, citrate), urine (PO_4, Ca).
   Increased blood PO_4.
   Irritability of nervous system, muscle twitch, tetany, death
   Cataracts

7. **Effects of Overdose, Excess**
   Increased blood (Ca, citrate, alkaline phosphatase), urine PO_4, demin-
     eralization of skeleton, osteoclast activity
   Decreased blood PO_4, muscle sensitivity
   Metastatic deposits of Ca in tissues, notably kidney

METABOLIC ROLE

1. **Biosynthesis**
   Precursors—17 of 20 standard amino acids. No Cys, Asn, or Gln
   Intermediates—No data
   Site(s) in cell—No data

2. **Production Sites:**   Parathyroid gland. Principal cells (?)

3. **Storage Areas:**   No data

4. **Blood Carriers:** α-globulin and albumin

5. **Half-life:**   20 min

6. **Target Tissues:**   Bone, kidney, muscle, mammary gland, gut

7. **Reactions:**   Reactive intermediate—Cyclic AMP—secondary messenger

Organ	Enzyme System	Effect
Bone and Kidney	Adenyl cyclase	Activated

8. **Mode of Action**
   Cellular
       Anabolic—No data
       Catabolic—Bone resorption
       Other
           Mitochondrial PO_4 increased

Mitochondrial swelling
Increased conversion pyruvate to citrate
Organismal
Raises renal Ca threshold
Lowers renal PO_4 threshold

9. **Catabolism**
Intermediates—Partial digestion in liver
Excretion Products—1% in urine

MISCELLANEOUS

1. **Relationship to Vitamins**
Vitamin D—Synergistic with PTH in maintenance of serum calcium

2. **Relationship to Other Hormones**
Estradiol—Synergises PTH in birds
Cortisol—Synergises PTH in vertebrates
T4, STH, Estradiol, Testosterone, Calcitonin—Antagonists to PTH

3. **Unusual Features**
Activity increased with molecular weight of analog
Demineralization of skeleton, formation of cysts with excess PTH
High citrate produced in bone action

4. **Possible Relationships of Deficiency Symptoms to Metabolic Action**
Decreased blood Ca, citrate—Lack of PTH mobilization of bone calcium
Increased blood PO_4—Urine threshold for PO_4 high without PTH
Irritability of nervous system—Decrease of blood calcium
Cataracts—?

28
Thyrocalcitonin

GENERAL INFORMATION

1. **Synonyms:** TCT, calcitonin

2. **History**
   1962—Copp discovered and named hormone with effects opposite to those of Parathormone
   1963—Munson extracted thyrocalcitonin from rat thyroids
   1964—Foster *et al.* reported that calcitonin originated in thyroid gland in goats
   1966—Pearse identified thyroid "C" cells as source of calcitonin

3. **Physiological Forms:** l-Thyrocalcitonin

4. **Active Analogs and Related Compounds:** No data

5. **Inactive Analogs and Related Compounds:** No data

6. **Antagonists:** Parathyroid hormone, vit. D

7. **Synergists:** Estradiol

8. **Physiological Functions**
   Decreases blood Ca [balances PTH (parathyroid hormone)]
   Inhibits bone resorption

Increases PO_4 excretion
Increases proline incorporation into bone

9. **Deficiency Diseases, Disorders:**   Medullary carcinoma of the thyroid (excess)

10. **Essentiality for Life:**   Not demonstrated

CHEMISTRY

1. **Structure**
   Polypeptide, 32 amino acids, synthesized
   Straight chain, one S–S ring: Porcine TCT Cys–Ser–Asn–Leu–Ser–
      Thr–Cys–Val–Leu–Ser–Ala–Try–Trp–Arg–Asn–Leu–Asn–
      Asn–Phe–His–Arg–Phe–Ser–Gly–Met–Gly–Phe–Gly–Pro–
      Glu–Thr–Pro

2. **Reactions**

Heat—Relatively stable	Oxidation—No data
Acid—Sol., Inactivates (conc.)	Reduction—No data
Alkali—Inactivates (conc.)	Light—No data
Water—Sol., acidic	Proteolysis—Pepsin and trypsin inactivates

3. **Properties**

Appearance—No data	Solubility
MW—3604	H_2O—Sol.
MP—No data	Acet., Alc.—Insol.
Crystal Form—No Data	Benz., Chl., Eth.—Insol.
Salts—No data	Absn. Max.—Approx 280 mμ
Important Groups for Activity	Chemical Nature—Acidic
S–S ring 1 + 7 position	polypeptide
Tyr and Try in	Misc.—pI = 4.8
positions 12 and 13	

4. **Commercial Production:**   Not available

5. **Isolation**
   Sources—Pork thyroid

Method

Extraction

(a) Extract with 0.2 *N* HCl 60-70°C for 5 min, filter after 1 hr

(b) Dialyze, pH 4.6, against 0.1 *M* acetate buffer at 4°C

(c) Precipitate from 1.5 *M* NaCl

Purification

(a) Gel filtration—Sephadex G-100, pH 4.6

(b) Ultrafiltration—If complexed to proteins earlier

6. **Determination**

Bioassay—Effect on plasma Ca level in rat

Physicochemical—Radioimmunoassay

MEDICAL AND BIOLOGICAL ROLE

1. **Species Occurrence, Specificity, and Antigenicity**

Occurrence—Found in most vertebrates

Specificity—High, great variation in interspecific potency

Antigenicity—Not antigenic

2. **Units**

MRC units or by weight

5-10 MRC milliunits lowers plasma Ca in rat by about 10%

3. **Normal Blood Levels:**   0.01 μg/100 ml plasma (rabbit)

4. **Administration**

Injection—Active

Topical—Inactive

Oral—Inactive

5. **Factors Affecting Release**

Inhibitors—No data

Stimulators—High plasma calcium level, glucagon

6. **Deficiency Symptoms:**   Blood Ca increase

7. **Effects of Overdose, Excess:**   Blood Ca decrease

METABOLIC ROLE

1. **Biosynthesis**
   Precursors—18 of 20 standard amino acids; Lys, Ile absent
   Intermediates—Unknown
   Site(s) in cell—Unknown

2. **Production Sites**
   Thyroid, parathyroid, and thymus (man)
   Parafollicular C cells derived from ultimobranchial body

3. **Storage Areas:**   Unknown

4. **Blood Carriers:**   Unknown

5. **Half-life:**   5-15 min (rabbit)

6. **Target Tissues:**   Bone, kidney, muscle

7. **Reactions**
   Reactive intermediate—Cyclic AMP—secondary messenger

Organ	Enzyme System	Effect
Thyroid	Adenyl cyclase	Activated
	Phosphorylase b	Activated

8. **Mode of Action**
   Cellular
   Anabolic—Increases proline incorporation into bone
   Catabolic—No data
   Other—No data
   Organismal
   Decreases blood calcium
   Inhibits bone resorption and citrate formation
   Increases PO_4 excretion
   Decreases glucose utilization and lactate production in bone

9. **Catabolism**
   Intermediates—Liver proteolysis
   Excretion products—Products of protein metabolism

MISCELLANEOUS

1. **Relationship to Vitamins:**   Vitamin D antagonizes TCT

2. **Relationship to Other Hormones**
     PTH—Antagonist to thyrocalcitonin
     Glucagon—Stimulates release of TCT
     Estradiol—Synergises and releases TCT

3. **Unusual Features:**   Birds have a gland separate from thyroid containing
        TCT

4. **Possible Relationships of Deficiency to Metabolic Action**
     Blood calcium increase—Unknown

29
Insulin

GENERAL INFORMATION

1. **Synonyms:**   None

2. **History**
   10 A.D.—Celsus described diabetic syndrome
   1899—Von Mering and Minkowski demonstrated relationship between pancreatectomy and diabetes mellitus
   1922—Macleod determined that islet cells produce insulin
   1922—Banting and Best prepared potent insulin extracts from dog pancreas
   1926—Abel *et al.* isolated crystalline insulin
   1955—Sanger *et al.* determined structure of insulin
   1966—Katsoyannis synthesized insulin (human and sheep)

3. **Physiological Forms:**   l-Insulin

4. **Active Analogs and Related Compounds:**   No data

5. **Inactive Analogs and Related Compounds**
   Oxidized, reduced insulin, proinsulin
   Alkali inactivated insulin

6. **Antagonists:**   Cortisol, glucagon, epinephrine, norepinephrine, STH (CHO and fat metabolism), T4

7. **Synergists:**   STH (protein metabolism), testosterone, estradiol

8. **Physiological Function**
     Regulates CHO and fat metabolism, esp. glucose and fat oxidations
     Stimulates amino acid and glucose transport into cells and protein
          synthesis
     Stimulates glycogen and mucopolysaccharide formation

9. **Deficiency Diseases, Disorders:**   Diabetes mellitus (faulty β-cells), azoturia,
          hyperlipemia, ketonemia

10. **Essentiality for Life:**   Essential for survival

CHEMISTRY

1. **Structure**
     Structure known and synthesized—51 amino acids
     Polypeptide, 2 parallel straight chains, -3— S—S bridges
     2 chains (ox insulin)
          α—21 amino acids—acidic: Gly—Ile—Val—Glu—Glu—
               Cys—Cys—Ala—Ser—Val—Cys—Ser—Leu—Tyr—Glu—Leu—Glu—
               Asp—Tyr—Cys—Asp
          β—30 amino acids—basic: Phe—Val—Asp—Glu—His—Leu—Cys—Gly—
               Ser—His—Leu—Val—Glu—Ala—Leu—Tyr—Leu—Val—Cys—Gly—
               Glu—Arg—Gly—Phe—Phe—Tyr—Thr—Pro—Lys—Ala

2. **Reactions**

Heat—Unstable	Oxidation—Inactivates
Acid—Stable	Reduction—Inactivates
Alkali—Inactivates	Light—No data
Water—Soluble, acidic	Proteolysis—Trypsin inactivates

3. **Properties**

Appearance—White crystalline powder	Important Groups for Activity
MW—5734 monomer	2 Disulfide bridges (S—S ring)
Polymer: 12,000-48,000, depending on pH	Active groups unknown
	Key positions—19-21 on α-chain; 22-30 on β-chain
MP—No data	Tyr, Asn
Crystal Form—Hexagonal system	
Salts—Zinc, Protamine	

Solubility
H$_2$O—Soluble
Acet., Alc.—Sol.
Benz., Chl., Eth.—Insol.

Absn. Max.—Approx. 280 mμ
Chemical Nature—Acidic
polypeptide
Misc.—pI = 5.3

4. Commercial Production: Extraction of beef or pork pancreas

5. Isolation

Sources—Pancreas—beef, pork
Method
Extract pancreas in 80% EtOH, pH 3 (H$_3$PO$_4$)
pH to 8 with NH$_4$OH precipitates impurities
Precipitate insulin with EtOH and ether
Dissolve in EtOH—H$_3$PO$_4$ buffer and precipitate insulin as picrate
Dissolve in acetone HCl
Precipitate with acetone
Wash and dry
Purification
Crystallize at pI in acetate buffer with 0.15-0.60% zinc
Precipitate with alc.
Salting out
Gel filtration and crystallization or electrophoresis

6. Determination

Bioassay
Isolated rat diaphragm; perfused heart; *in vitro* systems, for measuring glucose uptake
Lowering blood sugar in rabbit
Physicochemical
Radioimmunoassay
Immunoassay—Very sensitive for plasma insulin concentration

MEDICAL AND BIOLOGICAL ROLE

1. Species Occurrence, Specificity, and Antigenicity

Occurrence—Found in all vertebrates
Specificity—Moderate interspecific potency
Antigenicity—Moderate antigenicity. Pig and human sequence alike yet antigenic differences exist

2. Units: 1 I.U. = 1 USP unit = 0.04167 mg international standard

3. **Normal Blood Levels:** $0.1\text{-}3.0 \times 10^{-3}$ I.U./ml

4. **Administration**
   Injection—Subcutaneous
       Amorphous Insulin, Crystalline Insulin—Fact acting, short duration
       Protamine Insulin, Protamine Zn insulin—Slow, steady absorption
   Topical—Not used
   Oral
       Sulfonylureas—Stimulate secretion of insulin
       Hypoglycemic agents—Stimulate secretion of insulin
       Biguanides—Stimulate secretion of insulin

5. **Factors Affecting Release**
   Inhibitors
       Low blood sugar—Feedback
       Epinephrine
       Norepinephrine
   Stimulators
       High blood sugar—Feedback
       Elevated blood amino acid level
       Vagal stimulation
       Glucagon, ACTH, secretin, STH,
       Ketone bodies, sulfonylureas, biguanides
       Hypoglycemic agents
       Cortisol, T4

6. **Deficiency Symptoms**
   Polyphagia
   Decreases respiratory quotient
   Decreases tissue protein
   Polydipsia
   Hyperglycemia, Glycosuria—Underutilization and overproduction of
       glucose
   Polyurea
   Hyperlipemia
   Ketonemia
   Azoturia

7. **Effects of Overdose, Excess**
   Convulsions
   Increases glycogen storage
   Mental confusion

Coma
Headache
Tremor
Sweating
Apprehensiveness

METABOLIC ROLE

1. **Biosynthesis**
   Precursors—17 of 20 standard amino acids (aspartic acid, tryptophan, and methionine missing)
   Intermediates—Proinsulin
   Site(s) in cell—Unknown

2. **Production Sites:** β-cells of islets of pancreas

3. **Storage Areas:** β-granules in β-cells

4. **Blood Carriers:**   Circulating proteins; α,β-macroglobulins

5. **Half-life in Plasma:**   Nonlabeled insulin, < 9 min; insulin ^{131}I, 40 min

6. **Target Tissues:**   Systemic, esp. liver, adipose tissue, muscle, kidney.

7. **Reactions:**   Reactive form—unknown

Organ	Enzyme System	Effect
Liver	Lipase	Inhibited
	Adenyl cyclase	Inhibited
	Glycogen synthetase	Activated
Tissues	Hexokinase	Activated
	Phosphorylases	Activated

8. **Mode of Action**
   Cellular
   Anabolic—Increases mucopolysaccharide synthesis, protein synthesis, fatty acid synthesis, $_m$RNA synthesis
   Catabolic—Inhibits gluconeogenesis. Increases glucose oxidation
   Other—Increases transport glucose and A.A. across cell membrane (does not affect glucose entrance into hepatic cells, brain, blood cells). Inhibits cyclic AMP formation

Organismal

    Inhibits mobilization of fat from peripheral reservoirs

    Decreases blood (sugar, K, PO_4 ketones), liver gluconeogenesis, polyuria

    Increases liver and muscle glycogen, glucose absorption in gut, fat formation, nitrogen balance

9. **Catabolism**

    Intermediates—Insulinase in liver (antagonized by insulinase inhibitor)

    Excretion products—Metabolic products of amino acids

MISCELLANEOUS

1. **Relationship to Vitamins:** Vitamin C acts similarly to alloxan (i.e., antagonist)

2. **Relationship to Other Hormones**

    Cortisol, Glucagon, Epinephrine, Norepinephrine, T4, STH (CHO and fat metabolism)—Antagonistic to insulin

    Estradiol, Testosterone, STH (protein metabolism)—Synergistic with insulin

3. **Unusual Features**

    Contains 0.4% zinc in crystals

    First synthetic polypeptide hormone

    Multiple insulins in rat, bonito

    Forms fibrils when heated at low pH

    Antibody sites not identical with biological activity sites

    Frog—Pancreas not active until mid-metamorphosis

    Urodeles—Only β-cells in pancreas

    Vigorous exercise increases rate of transport of glucose into muscle cells even in absence of insulin

4. **Possible Relationships of Deficiency Symptoms to Metabolic Action**

    Hyperglycemia, decrease in respiratory quotient—Inability to metabolize and transport glucose into cells

    Hyperlipemia—Mobilization of fat from peripheral reserves

    Ketonemia—Incomplete oxidation of mobilized fat

    Azoturia (decrease in tissue protein)—Induced gluconeogenesis producing urea and ammonia

    Polydipsia—Thirst produced by glycosuria (polyuria)

    Polyphagia—Hunger produced by loss of urinary glucose

30
Glucagon

GENERAL INFORMATION

1. **Synonyms:** HGF, HG-Factor, hyperglycemic-glycogenolytic factor, glukagon

2. **History**
   1922—McLeod ⎫
   1923—Collip ⎬ Described hyperglycemic effect of pancreatic extracts
   1923—Kimball and Murlin suggested a second pancreatic hormone; named it glucagon
   1955—Staub, Sinn, and Behrens isolated and crystallized glucagon
   1956—Bromer *et al.* determined structure of glucagon
   1967—Wunsch synthesized glucagon

3. **Physiological Forms:** *l*-glucagon

4. **Active Analogs and Related Compounds:** Serotonin (G.I. tract, spleen, skin, tongue); isoproterenol, G.I. glucagon

5. **Inactive Analogs and Related Compounds:** UV-inactivated glucagon

6. **Antagonists:** Insulin

7. **Synergists:** Epinephrine (liver, muscle), norepinephrine, cortisol, cortisone

8. **Physiological Functions**

   Increases—Blood sugar, blood K^+, O_2 consumption, liver glycogenolysis, gluconeogenesis, nitrogen and salt excretion, glucose-1-P

   Decreases—Liver glycogen, protein formation, gastric juice, fatty acid synthesis

9. **Deficiency Diseases, Disorders:**   Hypoglycemic coma

10. **Essentiality for Life:**   Not essential for life of vertebrate organisms

CHEMISTRY

1. **Structure**

   Polypeptide (sequence determined): His—Ser—Glu—Gly—Thr—Phe—
   Thr—Ser—Asp—Tyr—Ser—Lys—Tyr—Leu—Asp—Ser—Arg—Arg—
   Ala—Glu—Asp—Phe—Val—Glu—Try—Leu—Met—Asp—Thr
   Straight single chain—His. - - - Thr., 29 amino acids
   No S—S bridges

2. **Reactions**

   Heat—Stable to 100°C
   Acid—Stable, pH 2
   Alkali—Stable, pH 9
   Water—Sol., basic

   Oxidation—No data
   Reduction—Stable to cysteine
     (removes contaminating
     insulin)
   Light—UV Inactivates
   Proteolysis—Leucine amino
     peptidase, pepsin, trypsin,
     chymotrypsin at pH = 6-8
     hydrolyze

3. **Properties**

   Appearance—White powder
   MW—3500 (29 A.A.)
   MP—No data
   Crystal Form—Rhombic
     dodecahedra
   Salts—HCl
   Important Groups for Activity
     Try, Met

   Solubility
     H_2O—Insol.
     Acet., Alc.—Insol.
     Benz., Chl., Eth.—Insol.
   Absn. Max.—278 mμ
   Chemical Nature—Basic polypeptide
   Misc.—pI = 7.5-8.5

4. **Commercial Production:**   Hog pancreas

5. Isolation
> Sources—Crude pork insulin
> Methods
>> Ppt. with acetone and salts at low pH
>> Crystallize from 0.033 M glycine buffer. pH 8.6 with 0.67 M urea
>> Purification: Starch zone electrophoresis

6. Determination
> Bioassay
>> Hyperglycemic response in cats
>> Glycogenolysis of liver slices
>> Reaction of phosphorylase in liver slices
> Physicochemical—Radioimmunoassay, immunoassay

MEDICAL AND BIOLOGICAL ROLE

1. **Species Occurrence, Specificity, and Antigenicity**
> Occurrence—Found in fish through mammals
> Specificity—Interspecies potency—Interreactive
> Antigenicity—Antigenic in rabbit or bovine x porcine glucagon, but not guinea pig glucagon

2. **Units:** By weight, also 1 I.U. = amount to increase blood sugar to 30 mg/100 ml

3. **Normal Blood Levels (Man):** 0.02-0.05 μg/100 ml plasma

4. **Administration**
> Injection—Glucagon HCl intravenous, intramuscular, or subcutaneous
>> Used to treat insulin-induced hypoglycemia
> Topical—Inactive
> Oral—Inactive

5. **Factors Affecting Release**
> Inhibitors—High blood sugar, $CoCl_2$ (α-cells)
> Stimulators—Hypoglycemia, fasting

6. **Deficiency Symptoms:** Low blood glucose

7. **Effects of Overdose:** Metaglucagon diabetes (destroy β-cells), increased food consumption, high blood glucose

METABOLIC ROLE

1. **Biosynthesis**

   Simple precursors—16 of standard 20 amino acids (no cysteine, isoleucine, proline, glutamic acid)

   Intermediates—Unknown

   Site(s) in cell—No data

2. **Production Sites**—α-cells in pancreas

3. **Storage Areas:**   Granules in α-cells

4. **Blood Carriers:**   Plasma proteins

5. **Half-life:**   Less than 10 min

6. **Target Tissues:**   Liver, adipose tissues, kidney

7. **Reactions**

   Reactive intermediate—Cyclic AMP—secondary messenger

Organ	Enzyme System	Effect
Liver	Glucokinase	Inhibited
	Glycogen synthetase	Inhibited
	Glycogenolysis enzymes	Activated
	Gluconeogenesis enzymes	Activated
	Adenyl cyclase	Activated
	Dephosphophosphorylase kinase	Activated
	Phosphorylase b	Activated
	Carbamoyl phosphate synthetase	Activated
	Argino-succinase	Activated
	Argino-succinic synthetase	Activated
Heart	Adenyl cyclase	Activated

8. **Mode of Action**

   Cellular

   Anabolic—No data

   Catabolic

   Decreased protein and fatty acid synthesis

   Increased lipolysis

   Increased CHO glycogenolysis

   Increased protein catabolism

   Other

   Increased cyclic AMP formation

   Decreased adrenal ascorbic acid

Organismal
Stimulates hepatic glycogenolysis and gluconeogenesis
Increases adipose tissue lipolysis
Stimulates release of catecholamines by adrenal medulla
Increases nitrogen K, Na, Cl, PO_4 excretion
Increases blood sugar, ketone bodies
Decreases gastric juice flow
Increases heart rate, ventricular contractility
Decreases atrio-ventricular conduction time
Retards G.I. contractions

9. Catabolism
Intermediates—Proteolysis in liver, kidney, blood—glucagonase (protease), recycling
Excretion products—End products of protein metabolism (urea, CO_2)

MISCELLANEOUS

1. Relationship to Vitamins
Vitamin C—Depletion of adrenal ascorbic acid by glucagon

2. Relationship to Other Hormones
Epinephrine, Norepinephrine—Secretion stimulated by glucagon, also synergistic
Cortisol, Cortisone—Synergistic to glucagon
Insulin—Antagonistic to glucagon

3. Unusual Features
Tissue differences in glucagon response
More conc. in female than male pancreas
G.I. glucagon not identical with pancreatic glucagon
Traces of heavy metals (Cu, Co) found in glucagon preparations

4. Possible Relationships of Deficiency Symptoms to Metabolic Action
Low blood glucose—lack of glucose-releasing activity by glucagon into plasma

31
Aldosterone

GENERAL INFORMATION

1. **Synonyms:** Electrocortin, mineralocorticoid, aldocortin, 18-oxocorticosterone

2. **History**
   - 1953—Simpson *et al.* ⎫ Isolated crystalline aldosterone
   - 1954—Mattox *et al.* ⎭ from adrenals
   - 1954—Wettstein and Anner devised highly sensitive test for mineralocorticoid activity
   - 1954—Simpson *et al.* determined structure of aldosterone
   - 1955—Schmidlin *et al.* synthesized dl-aldosterone
   - 1956—Vischer *et al.* synthesized d-aldosterone
   - 1956—Neher and Wettstein isolated 15 more steroids similar to aldosterone and cortisol

3. **Physiological Forms:** Hemiacetal form (11,18-semiacetal), aldehyde form

4. **Active Analogs and Related Forms** (Mineralocorticoids)
   Natural—11-Deoxycorticosterone, corticosterone
   Synthetic—2α-Methylcortisol, 9α-fluorocortisol, 2α-methyl-9α-fluorocortisol

5. **Inactive Analogs and Related Forms (for Aldosterone Function):** Cortexolone, dexamethasone, prednisolone

6. **Antagonists**

 Natural—Cortisol, pineal factor, estradiol, progesterone, vasopressin (kidney), prostaglandins

 Synthetic—3-Spironolactone, aldactone-A

7. **Synergists:** 11-deoxycorticosterone, vasopressin, oxytocin, angiotensin II, renin, STH

8. **Physiological Functions**

 Maintenance of normal electrolyte blood balance

 Prolongs survival of adrenalectomized animals

 Accelerates gluconeogenesis

 Regulates kidney function

9. **Deficiency Diseases, Disorders:** Addison's disease, (deficiency), Cushing's syndrome (excess), adrenocortical insufficiency, primary hyperaldosteronism

10. **Essentiality for Life:** One of the most essential of all hormones. Absence can be fatal in short time period

CHEMISTRY

1. **Structure**

Aldosterone (aldehyde form), $C_{21}H_{28}O_5$

2. **Reactions**

Heat—Stable

Acid—Decomposes

Alkali—Fluoresces (conc.)

 Isomerizes to 17-iso-aldosterone

Water—Slightly sol.

Oxidation—Loses aldehyde group

Reduction—Unstable

Light—Stable

3. Properties

Appearance—Colorless crystals
MW—360.4
MP—164°C
Crystal Form—Needles (acetate)
Salts, Esters—Acetate
Important Groups for Activity
   —C(18)HO
   —C(21)H$_2$OH
   —C(11)OH

Solubility
   H$_2$O—Sparingly
   Acet., Alc.—Sol.
   Benz., Chl., Eth.—Sol.
   Absn. Max.—240 mμ
Chemical Nature
   Hemiacetal, aldehyde
   Alc., ketone—Reducing steroid
   α_D^{23} = +145 (acet.)

4. Commercial Production: Microbiological (stereospecific hydroxylation)

5. Isolation

Sources: Beef adrenal extract
Methods
  (1) Partition aqueous extract with pentane-methanol
  (2) Chromatograph on kieselguhr, elute with petroleum ether-benzene-CHCl$_3$
  (3) Rechromatograph on powdered cellulose, elution with toluene-petroleum ether-methanol
  (4) Recrystallize from methanol

6. Determination

Bioassay
   Life maintenance in adrenalectomized animals
   Increase muscular work performance
   Cold stress reactions on adrenalectomy
   In vitro incubation of perfused tissues
Physicochemical—Monitor Na/K ratios in urine

MEDICAL AND BIOLOGICAL ROLE

1. Species Occurrence, Specificity, and Antigenicity

Occurrence: All vertebrate species studied, except cyclostomes
Specificity: Same electrolyte regulator, all species
Antigenicity: None reported

2. Units: mg or μg

3. Normal Blood Levels (Man): 0.03 μg/100 ml

4. **Administration**
   Injection—Main route
   Topical—No reports
   Oral—Active

5. **Factors Affecting Release**
   Inhibitors
   Decreased K^+ in blood
   Increased Na^+ in blood
   Hemodilution
   Stimulators
   Angiotensin II—Renin
   Stress, decreased Na^+, decreased blood vol.
   Pregnancy
   ACTH (slightly)
   Increased blood pressure in carotid arteries
   Increased K^+ in blood

6. **Deficiency Symptoms (Humans)**
   Decreased—Blood (pressure, sugar, pH), weight, liver glycogen, urinary
   K^+, temperature, reproductive functions
   Increased—Urinary (Na^+, Cl^-, HCO_3^-)
   Kidney failure, muscular weakness, GI disturbances, hemoconcentration,
   stress intolerance, acidosis

7. **Effects of Overdose, Excess**
   Hypertension
   Congestive heart failure
   Increased Na^+ and H_2O in blood, muscles
   Hemodilution
   Hypokalemia
   Edema
   Alkalosis
   Diabetes insipidus (type of)

METABOLIC ROLE

1. **Biosynthesis:**   Acetate $\to$ Mevalonate $\to$ Squalene $\to$ Cholesterol $\to$ Pregnenolone $\to$ Progesterone $\to$ Aldosterone
   Site(s) in Cell—Membranes

2. **Production Sites:**   Adrenal cortex (zona glomerulosa), embryonic rest cells

3. **Storage Areas:**   None

4. **Blood Carriers**
   Lipoproteins, albumin
   Conjugates, Free Steroid—Combined with above proteins

5. **Half-life:**   25 min

6. **Target Tissues:**   Distal renal tubules, sweat and salivary glands, intestinal mucosa, gills (fish), skin (amphibia), nasal gland (bird), rectal gland (sharks)

7. **Reactions**
   Reactive form—Equilibrium (hemiacetal-aldehyde) redox couple

Organ	Enzyme System	Effect
Kidney	1. Unknown enzymes involved in sodium transport	Activated
	2. Also enzymes similar to cortisol (glucocorticoid function)	Activated
	3. RNA polymerase	Activated
Liver, muscle, plasma, general	Similar to cortisol; see Cortisol	Activated

8. **Mode of Action**
   Cellular
   Anabolic—Liver (proteins, CHO, nucleic acids)
   Catabolic—Extrahepatic (proteins, fats, CHO, nucleic acids)
   Other—Increases Na^+ active transport in renal tubules, activates redox pump, H_2O transported with Na^+
   Organismal
   Increases blood Na^+, volume, pressure; urinary K^+, H^+; cold tolerance, muscle work performance, liver glycogen
   Decreases blood K^+, H^+; urine Na^+, H_2O, volume; eosinophils, lymphocytes

9. **Catabolism**
   Intermediates—Tetrahydro derivative (inactive)
   Excretion Products—30-40% Glucuronides, 4-8% free, 52-66% other conjugates

MISCELLANEOUS

1. **Relationship to Vitamins**

    Vitamin C—Adrenal cortex depleted of vit. C on production of aldosterone

    Niacin—NADPH involved in synthesis of aldosterone

    Biotin—Prolongs life in adrenalectomized rats

2. **Relationship to Other Hormones**

    Cortisol—Synergistic to aldosterone in glucocorticoid activity; antagonistic to aldosterone in water metabolism

    ACTH—Trigger for small release of aldosterone

    Vasopressin, Oxytocin—Synergists for aldosterone action in water metabolism

    Angiotensin II, Renin—Stimulate production of aldosterone

    Other hormones antagonistic or synergistic with cortisol (glucocorticoid action)—*see* Cortisol

3. **Unusual Features**

    Not a glucocorticoid even though it has —OH on C-11 and 1/3 of glucocorticoid power of cortisol

    Redox couple—Hemiacetal-aldehyde equilibrium

    No nervous controls

    Active on oral administration

    Most water soluble of all steroids

    Largely independent of ACTH control

4. **Possible Relationships of Deficiency Symptoms to Metabolic Action**

    Loss of mineralocorticoid functions. Failure of sodium pump and sodium-water reabsorption mechanisms in kidney tubules

    Increased—Urinary (Na^+, Cl^-, HCO_3^-). Decreased urinary K^+, blood pH and pressure

    Acidosis, kidney failure

    Hemoconcentration

    Weight loss

    Loss of glucocorticoid functions; decreased gluconeogenesis

    Muscular weakness

    G.I. disturbances

    Stress intolerance

    Decreased blood sugar

    Decreased liver glycogen

    Decreased temperature

32
Cortisol

GENERAL INFORMATION

1. **Synonyms:** Hydrocortisone, Compound F, 17-hydroxycorticosterone, Substance M

2. **History**
   1937—Reichstein isolated cortisol from adrenal glands
   1942—Von Euw, Reichstein determined configuration of cortisol
   1948—Mason, Sprague isolated cortisol from urine
   1950—Reich *et al.* isolated cortisol from blood
   1950—Wendler *et al.* synthesized cortisol
   1951—Zaffaroni *et al.* demonstrated biosynthesis of cortisol in adrenals

3. **Physiological Forms:** Cortisol, cortisone

4. **Active Analogs and Related Compounds (Glucocorticoids)**
   Natural—Deoxycorticosterone, cortexolone, cortisone ("E"), corticosterone ("B"), dehydrocorticosterone ("A")
   Synthetic—Dexamethasone, 9α-F-cortisol, prednisone, prednisolone

5. **Inactive Analogs and Related Compounds:** Estrone, progesterone, 17-α-hydroxyprogesterone, cortexolone, adrenosterone

6. **Antagonists:** Protein and CHO metabolism—Insulin; STH, estrogens, testosterone

7. **Synergists:**   Fat metabolism—STH; epinephrine, norepinephrine, PTH, T4

8. **Physiological Functions**

   Increases—Protein catabolism (exc. liver) gluconeogensis, carbohydrate anabolism (liver), blood sugar, glucose absorption, brain
   excitation, spread of infections, urinary glucose and nitrogen, stress
   tolerance, lactation, water diuresis

   Decreases—Fat anabolism, growth rate, inflammation, eosinophils, lymphocytes, antigen sensitivity, respiratory quotient, ketosis, wound
   healing, skin pigmentation, RBC hemolysis

   Regulates—General adaptation syndrome, water balance, blood pressure,
   hormone release

9. **Disorders and Deficiency Diseases:**   Addison's disease (deficiency),
   Cushing's syndrome (excess), adrenal insufficiency, adrenogenital
   syndrome, rheumatic arthritis, inflammation

10. **Essentiality for Life:**   Absence causes shortening of life span due to
    inability to respond to stress situations

CHEMISTRY

1. **Structure:**

Cortisol, $C_{21}H_{30}O_5$

2. **Reactions**

Heat—Oxidizes	Oxidation—Forms cortisone
Acid—Esterifies	C-11 Hydroxyl $\rightarrow$ Keto
Fluorescent in H_2SO_4 (conc.)	Reduction—Stable
Alkali—Stable (dilute)	Light—Stable
Fluorescent (conc.)	
Water—very sl. sol.	

3. **Properties**

Appearance—White powder
MW—362.5
MP—217-220°C
Crystal Form—Rectilinear
  plates
Salts, Esters—
  Acetate
Important Groups for Activity
  —C(17)OH
  —C(11)OH
  —C(21)H$_2$OH

Solubility
  H$_2$O—0.28 mg/ml
  Acet., Alc.—15, 6.2 mg/ml
  Chl., Eth.—9.3, 0.35 mg/ml
  Absn. Max.—242 mμ
Chemical Nature
  Reducing agent
  Alcohol, ketone
  $\alpha_D^{22} = 167$ (EtOH)

4. **Commercial Production:** Extraction and isolation from beef and hog adrenals

5. **Isolation**

Sources—Adrenal cortex
Methods
  Free
    Extract with dil. alkali, partition between 2 solvents
    Chromatography—Glass, paper, thin layer, gas, liquid
    Columns—Florasil
    Countercurrent distribution
  Conjugates—Extract tissue, paper chromatography, alumina columns

6. **Determination**

Bioassay:
  Increased—Liver glycogen, lifespan in cold, tolerance to trauma, isotope uptake.
  Decreased—Eosinophils, lymphocytes
Physicochemical
  Reduction to red formazan
  Oxidation to 17-oxosteroids
  Phenylhydrazone formation
  Fluorescence at 550 or 570 mμ
  Polarography

MEDICAL AND BIOLOGICAL ROLE

1. **Species Occurrence, Specificity, and Antigenicity**
   Occurrence—Cortisol major form of glucocorticoids in primates, dog,
       fish, decreasing in activity in lower forms. Corticosterone major
       glucocorticoid in rodents, birds, amphibians, reptiles
   Specificity—Can cross species lines without loss of activity
   Antigenicity—Not antigenic

2. **Units:**   By weight, μg

3. **Normal Blood Levels:**   10 μg/100 ml (man)

4. **Administration**
   Injection—Intramuscular
   Oral—Active. Prednisone form used
   Topical—Acetonides in creams, lotions

5. **Factors Affecting Release**
   Inhibitors
       Pituitary hypofunction
       Diurnal rhythm—Low in afternoon
       Decreased ACTH
       Increased plasma-glucocorticoids
   Stimulators
       Pregnancy, infancy, stress
       ACTH ingestion and ACTH increase
       Adrenal hyperfunction
       Angiotensin II, insulin, estrogens
       Glucagon, vasopressin
       Decreased plasma glucocorticoids

6. **Deficiency Symptoms (Humans)**
   Decreased
       Growth, secondary sex characteristics
       Blood pressure, body temperature
       Kidney function, leading to death
       Liver glycogen, gluconeogenesis
       Intestinal absorption, blood sugar
       Stress response—ultimately death
   Increased
       Glucose oxidation, ACTH levels, respiratory quotient

Fat anabolism, hemoconcentration
Muscular weakness
Skin pigmentation
Insulin sensitivity

7. **Effects of Overdose (Excess)**
Buffalo obesity, bruisability, moon-face
Osteoporosis (demineralization of bone)
Adrenal regression
Anesthesia
Atherosclerosis, hypercholesterolemia, lipemia
Diabetes
Alkalosis
Decreased growth
Inhibition of inflammatory responses and wound healing

METABOLIC ROLE

1. **Biosynthesis:**   Acetate $\rightarrow$ Mevalonate $\rightarrow$ Squalene $\rightarrow$ Cholesterol
$\rightarrow$ Pregnenolone $\rightarrow$ Progesterone $\rightarrow$ 17α-Hydroxyprogesterone
$\rightarrow$ Cortisol
Sites in cell—Mitochondria, microsomes

2. **Production Sites:**   Adrenal cortex, placenta, embryonic rest cells

3. **Storage:**   Adrenal cortex (small amount)

4. **Blood Carriers:**   Lipoproteins, conjugates, α-globulins (transcortin), albumin; also free

5. **Half-life:**   1½-3 hr

6. **Target Tissues:**   Liver, central nervous system, hypothalamus, thymus, lymph nodes, intestine, connective tissues, skin, mammary gland, vascular system, general systemic

7. **Reactions**
Reactive Form: Cortisol $\rightleftharpoons$ cortisone (redox couple)

Enzyme Systems:

Organ	Enzyme Systems	Effect
Liver	Phosphoenolpyruvate carboxykinase	Activated
	Pyruvate carboxylase	Activated
	Tryptophan pyrrolase	Activated
	Glycolytic cycle enzymes	Activated
	Krebs cycle enzymes	Activated
	Urea cycle enzymes	Activated
	Deaminases and transaminases	Activated
Liver, kidney	Glucose-6-phosphatase	Activated
	Glycogen synthetase	Activated
	Arginase	Activated
Liver, plasma	Alkaline phosphatase	Activated
Muscle	Aminopeptidase	Activated
General	Histidine decarboxylase	Inhibited
	Hexokinase	Inhibited

8. Mode of Action

Cellular

Anabolic—Increases liver (protein, nucleic acid, CHO, fat) synthesis

Catabolic—Increases extrahepatic (protein, lipid, and nucleic acid) breakdown; decreases extrahepatic CHO breakdown

Other—Redox mechanisms maintained; water and sodium membrane transport regulated in kidney glomerulus (with aldosterone)

Organismal

Maintains circulation and blood pressure (with aldosterone)

Maintains fluid balance (with aldosterone)

Maintains renal function (with aldosterone)

Releases other hormones

Maintains stress reactions

Regulates ACTH output of pituitary

Maintains collagen, capillary permeability

9. Catabolism

Intermediates—Bile salts, 17-hydroxy steroids

Excretion products

Urine

100 (approx.) different steroids in urine

87% Glucuronides or sulfates—Cortols, cortolones, 17-hydroxy steroids

4% Free metabolites—Cortols, cortolones, 17-hydroxy steroids

1% Free cortisol—Cortols, cortolones, 17-hydroxy steroids

Feces—Bile salt derivatives

MISCELLANEOUS

1. Relationship to Vitamins

Vitamin C—May be needed for steroid hormone biosynthesis; depleted from adrenal cortex on cortical secretion

Niacin—NADPH required for steroid hormone biosynthesis

Vitamin D—Action antagonized by cortisol, i.e., reduces Ca absorption in intestine

Pantothenic acid, folic acid maintain secretions of steroids by adrenal cortex

Biotin—Adrenocortical insufficiency noted in biotin deficiency

Vitamin A—Deficiency of vitamin A causes cortical necrosis

2. Relationship to Other Hormones

Estradiol-17β—Antagonist to cortisol protein metabolic effects

Insulin—Antagonist to cortisol (CHO, protein, lipid) metabolic effects

STH—Antagonist to cortisol protein metabolic effects

Testosterone—Antagonist to cortisol protein metabolic effects

Cortisone—Converted to cortisol in body (redox couple)

T4, Norepinephrine, Epinephrine—Potentiated by cortisol, synergistic

ACTH—Production stopped via feedback mechanism of cortisol

PTH—Synergist to cortisol in bone resorption

Vasopressin, Oxytocin—Antagonist to cortisol water balance effects, stimulants for production of glucocorticoids

Glucagon—Stimulant for production of cortical hormones

3. Unusual Features

Production of euphoria, anesthetic action

Decreased activity if side chain is lengthened

Substituents on C-20, C-18, determine antihemolytic activity

Suppression of mast cell activity, migration of lymphocytes and phagocytes

Inhibition of wound healing and collagen formation by fibroblasts

Inhibition of antibody production, regression of thymus tissue

Suppresses mitosis in lymphoid tissue

Species difference in sensitivity

4. Possible Relationships of Deficiency Symptoms to Metabolic Action

Osteoporosis—Antagonism to vit. D; synergism with PTH

Diabetes—Inhibition of glucose oxidation

Alkalosis—Retention of sodium

Bruisability—Depletion of vit. C (?)

Buffalo obesity, Moon-face—Antagonism to insulin (?)
Adrenal regression—Shut-off of ACTH production
Anesthesia—Effects on membranes (?)
Atherosclerosis—Diabetogenic effect (?)

33
Estradiol

GENERAL INFORMATION

1. **Synonyms:** Estradiol-17β, female hormone, β-estradiol, dihydrotheelin, dihydrofollicular hormone, dihydrofolliculin

2. **History**
   1929—Doisy, Butenandt, *et al.* isolated and crystallized estrone from pregnancy urine
   1930—Marrian isolated estriol from pregnancy urine
   1932—Marrian, Butenandt determined structure of estrone and estriol
   1936—McCorquodale isolated crystalline estradiol from pregnancy urine and sow ovaries
   1940—Inhoffen synthesized estradiol from cholesterol
   1948—Anner and Miescher totally synthesized estrone

3. **Physiological Forms:** Estrone, estriol, estradiol (Estrogens)

4. **Active Analogs and Related Compounds** (Estrogens)
   Synthetic—Diethylstilbesterol, hexestrol, dienestrol, benzestrol, ethinyl-estradiol, chlorotrianisene
   Natural—Estriol, estrone, equilin

5. **Inactive Analogs and Related Compounds** (Estrogen function)
   Pregnanediol, lumiestrone, progesterone, 17α-estradiol, 17α-hydroxy-progesterone, 17α-hydroxypregnenolone

6. **Antagonists:**   Progesterone, cortisol, testosterone (all concentration dependent); uterine factor, melatonin, ethamoxytriphetol, aldosterone

7. **Synergists:**   Prolactin, progesterone, androgens, corticoids, STH, oxytocin, T4, relaxin, insulin

8. **Physiological Functions**
   Regulates menstrual cycle, female sex behavior
   Maintains secondary sex characteristics
   Affects antibody properties
   Induces estrus, uterine hypertrophy, vaginal cornification, potentiates and stimulates calcitonin secretion

9. **Deficiency Diseases, Disorders:**   Menopause (natural deficiency) gonadal dysgenesis, delayed maturation

10. **Essentiality for Life:**   Not for life of organism, but for reproduction of organism

CHEMISTRY

1. **Structure**

Estradiol-17β, $C_{18}H_{24}O_2$

2. **Reactions**

Heat—Stable	Oxidation—Unstable. Forms
Acid—Stable (dilute)	estriol or estrone
Fluoresces (conc.)	Reduction—Unstable
Alkali—Sol., stable	Light—No data
Water—Insol.	

3. **Properties**

Appearance—colorless powder	MP—173-179°C
MW—272.4	Crystal Form—Prisms

Salts, Esters—Acetate,
  benzoate, propionate,
  heptanoate, valerate
Important Groups for Activity
  Aromatic Ring A
  $-C(3)OH, -C(17)OH$

Solubility
  H_2O—Insol.
  (Estriol—3 mg/100 cc H_2O)
  Acet., Alc.—Sol.
  Benz., Chl., Eth.—Sol.
  Absn. Max.—225, 280 mμ
  Chemical Nature—Alcohol,
    aromatic, phenolic
  $\alpha_D^{22} = 76\text{-}83$

4. **Commercial Production**
  Extract pregnant mare's urine
  Total synthesis

5. **Isolation**
  Sources—Pregnancy urine of mares, follicular liquor of sow ovaries
  Method
    Protein-bound or conjugated steroids: 15% HCl, 60 min 100°C, or
      sephadex G-25 with H_2O elution, or amberlite column LA-2,
      elution with ethyl acetate at pH = 2; saponification
    Free steroids: ether extraction
  Purification
    Countercurrent distribution
    Column chromatography
    High-voltage electrophoresis

6. **Determination**
  Bioassay
    Vaginal cornification
    Increase in uterine weight in ovariectomized animals
    Topical application in vagina; vaginal smear of exfoliated cells
  Physicochemical
    Fluorescence assay
    Colorimetry—Kober reaction
    Chromatography
    Radioimmunoassay

MEDICAL AND BIOLOGICAL ROLE

1. **Species Occurrence, Specificity, Antigenicity**
  Occurrence—All vertebrates, but different distribution of activities for
    three physiological forms. Some plants

Specificity
 17β-Estradiol, estrone (human, dog, pig, rat)
 Estrone, equilin, equilinin (horse)
 17α-Estradiol (sheep, goat, beef)
 17-Epiestriol (mouse)
 Species difference in sensitivity
Antigenicity—No antigenicity reported

2. **Units:** 1 mg = 10,000 I.U.

3. **Normal Blood Levels (Man):** Male .008 μg/100 ml (estradiol and estrone). Females 0.2 μg/100 ml or less (estrone and estriol). Pregnant Females (av.) 2.1 μg/100 ml estradiol, 6.5 μg/100 ml estrone, 10.9 μg/100 ml estriol (varies with stage of pregnancy)

4. **Administration:**
 Injection—Subcutaneous, intramuscular
 Topical—In creams and cosmetics
 Oral—Inactive free form. Active as esters or synthetic analogs. Various synthetic estrogens used in small quantity with synthetic progestogens in contraceptive pills

5. **Factors Affecting Release**
 Inhibitors—Feedback via blood to hypothalamus
 Stimulators—FSH and LH (cyclic via hypothalamus)

6. **Deficiency Symptoms (Humans)**
 Delayed maturation
 Female accessory and reproductive organs regress
 Decreased female behavioral pattern
 Senescence
 Menopause

7. **Effects of Overdose, Excess**
 Tumors
 Inhibition of gonads (decrease FSH, LH) $\rightarrow$ permanent sterility

METABOLIC ROLE

1. **Biosynthesis:** Acetate $\rightarrow$ Mevalonate $\rightarrow$ Squalene $\rightarrow$ Cholesterol $\rightarrow$ Pregnenolone $\rightarrow$ Progesterone $\rightarrow$ 17α-Hydroxyprogesterone $\rightarrow$ Androstenedione $\rightarrow$ Testosterone $\rightarrow$ 19-Hydroxytestosterone $\rightarrow$ Estradiol
 Site(s) in cell—Mitochondria, microsomes

2. **Production Sites**
   All vertebrates
   Ovarian follicles (membrane granulosa, theca interna)
   Testes (interstitial cells)
   Corpus luteum, adrenal cortex (fasciculata reticularis)
   Placenta, embryonic rest cells

3. **Storage Areas:**   Unknown

4. **Blood Carriers**
   Plasma proteins—Estriol glucuronides, free estrone and estradiol
   Plasma lipoprotein, estroprotein, serum albumin, red cell proteins

5. **Half-life:**   2-4 min

6. **Target Tissues:**   Systemic; uterus, mammary gland, vagina, ovary (corpus
   luteum), secondary female sex organs, skin, CNS, thyroid, thymus,
   long bones, anterior pituitary, hypothalamus

7. **Reactions**
   Reactive forms (Redox couple)
   Estradiol $\rightleftharpoons$ estrone $\rightarrow$ estriol (oxidation product)

Organ	Enzyme System	Effect
Uterus	Lactic acid dehydrogenase	Activated
	Phosphorylase b $\rightarrow$ a	Activated
	RNA polymerase	Activated
Placenta	Isocitric dehydrogenase	Activated
Endometrium	Glucose-6-phosphate dehydrogenase	Activated
Kidney	Kynurenine aminotransferase	Inhibited
Liver	Kynureninase	Inhibited
	N^1-Methylnicotinamide oxidase	Inhibited

8. **Mode of Action**
   Cellular
   Anabolic
   RNA and protein synthesis (uterus) increased
   CHO synthesis (uterus) increased
   Increased growth (uterus)
   Catabolic—CHO glycolysis (uterus) increased
   Other
   Direct action on nucleus

Increases mitosis (uterus)
Transcription of RNA affected
Hyperpolarization of cell membranes
Organismal
Uterus
Increases glycolysis, respiration, H_2O permeability, hyperemia
Releases histamine
Potentiates and stimulates TCT in calcium bone deposition
Development of female characteristics
Growth of female $1°$ and $2°$ sex organs
Estradiol, estrone—Act on corpus luteum
Estriol—Acts on sex organs
Regulates menstrual cycle and sex behavior
Maintains secondary sex characteristics
Affects antibody properties

9. Catabolism
Intermediates—Estriol
Excretion Products

Urine—Mainly conjugated $\dfrac{\text{estrone glucuronide or } SO_4}{\text{estriol glucuronide or } SO_4} = 1/3$

Free—As estriol or 16-epiestriol
Pregnancy—Estrone + estradiol increases 100x. Estriol increases 1000x
Feces—Enterohepatic circulation of estrogens

MISCELLANEOUS

1. Relationship to Vitamins
Folic acid—Involved in mitotic effect of estradiol
Niacin (TPN)(DPN)—Involved in increased respiration and in cholesterol precursor synthesis
Vitamin E—Involved in gonadotropin production or release
Vitamin B_6—Competes as cofactor with estrogen sulfate in kynurenine aminotransferase activity
Vitamin D—Synergistic in calcium metabolism with estradiol

2. Relationship to Other Hormones
Progesterone, Cortisol, Testosterone—Antagonistic or synergistic to estradiol depending on relative concentrations of estradiol and other hormone

Prolactin, STH, Oxytocin, T4, Relaxin—Synergistic to estradiol
TCT—Potentiated and stimulated by estradiol
FSH, LH—Stimulate release or production of estradiol

3. Unusual Features

Estradiol-17$\beta \rightleftharpoons$ estrone $\rightarrow$ estriol (activity 1000:100:1)
Aromatic ring—Carcinogenicity implicated
Redox couple estradiol $\rightleftharpoons$ estrone
Derived from testosterone in biosynthesis
Occurrence of estrogens in plants—Genistein, Coumestrol (active)
Tumor formation enhanced by estradiol
Enterohepatic circulation of estradiol
Variable species forms
Synthetic estrogens not steroids

4. Possible Relationships of Deficiency to Metabolic Action

Ovarian regression—Decrease of mitosis in sex tissues
Regression of female sex organs and secondary sex characteristics—
decrease of mitosis in sex tissues
Decreased female sex behavior patterns—Decrease of estradiol in central
nervous system.
Senescence, menopause—Decrease in mitosis in sex organs

34
Progesterone

GENERAL INFORMATION

1. Synonyms: Progestin, luteosterone, corpus luteum hormone

2. History

1903—Fraenkel demonstrated that removal of corpora lutea in pregnant rabbits terminates pregnancy, prevents attachment of ovum to uterus

1928—Corner and Allen restored progestational changes in above rabbits with extracts of corpora lutea

1930—Fels and Slotta ⎫
1932—Allen   ⎬ Obtained crude crystalline concentrates
1932—Fevold and Hisaw ⎭ containing progestational activity

1934—Butenandt et al. ⎫
    Slotta et al.   ⎬ Isolated pure crystalline
    Allen et al.   ⎬ corpus luteum hormone
    Hartmann et al.   ⎭

1934—Slotta et al. proposed formula for corpus luteum hormone

1934—Butenandt, Fernholz synthesized progesterone from stigmasterol

3. Physiological Forms: Progesterone, 17α-Hydroxyprogesterone

4. Active Analogs and Related Compounds: (Progestins, progestogens)
Natural
    20α-Hydroxypregnenone

222

20β-Hydroxypregnenone
11-Dehydroprogesterone
Cortexone
17α-Hydroxyprogesterone
Synthetic
A-Norprogesterone
19-Norprogesterone
21-Norprogesterone
Ethisterone
17α-Methyltestosterone
6α-Methyl-17α-acetoxyprogesterone
Δ^1-Dehydro-6α-methyl-17α-acetoxyprogesterone

5. **Inactive Analogs and Related Compounds**
5α-Pregnane-3β-ol-20-one, 21-ethylprogesterone
11β-Hydroxyprogesterone, pregnanediol, pregnanetriol

6. **Antagonists:**   (Estradiol, testosterone, oxytocin, aldosterone) all concentration dependent

7. **Synergists:**   Estradiol, prolactin, testosterone, cortisol, STH, T4, relaxin, oxytocin

8. **Physiological Functions**
Low concentrations
Prepare uterus for blastocyst implantation, promote ovulation and mammary gland development
Regulate female sex accessory organs, weak corticosteroid properties, precursor to sex hormones
Higher concentrations
Maintain pregnancy, repress ovulation and sex activity, inhibit vaginal cornification, and parturition, decrease myometrial excitation

9. **Deficiency Diseases, Disorders:**   Pseudopregnancy (laboratory animals), acne, dysfunctional uterine bleeding

10. **Essentiality for Life**
Indirectly essential for life via corticosteroid requirement
Essential for aldosterone and glucocorticoid formation
Essential for reproduction in female vertebrates

CHEMISTRY

Structure

Progesterone, $C_{21}H_{30}O_2$

2. Reactions

Heat—Stable
Acid—Unstable; fluoresces
in H_2SO_4
Alkali—Unstable
Water—Insol.

Oxidation—Unstable
Reduction—Unstable;
reduces to pregnanediol
Light—Unstable

3. Properties

Appearance—white powder
MW—314.5
MP—$\alpha = 128°C$
$\beta = 121°C$
Crystal Form
α-Orthorhombic prisms
β-Orthorhombic needles
Salts, Esters-Acetate,
caproate
Important Groups for Activity
—C(3)=O,
—C(4)=C(5)—
—C(20)—CH$_3$
$\overset{\|}{O}$

Solubility
H_2O—Insol.
Acet., Alc.—Sol.
Benz., Chl., Eth.—Sol.
Absn. Max.—240 mμ
Chemical Nature
Ketone, steroid
$\alpha_D = 172\text{-}182$ (dioxane)

4. Commercial Production

Synthesis from cholesterol, stigmasterol, or diosgenin
Isolation from sow ovary corpora lutea

5. Isolation

Sources—Sow ovary corpora lutea

Methods

Extract with alkali

Extract with ether or ether-ethanol (1:3) or methyl acetate-benzene

Partition between hexane (or petroleum ether) and 70% methyl alcohol

Purify by chromatography: celite column, thin layer, paper or counter current distribution

6. **Determination**

Bioassay

Decidual responses

Change of progesterone in endometrium

Physicochemical

Absorption at 240 mμ or at 290 mμ in H_2SO_4

Yellow fluorescence with $SbCl_3$

Blue absorption with phosphomolybdic acid

Protein-binding assay

MEDICAL AND BIOLOGICAL ROLE

1. **Species Occurrence, Specificity, Antigenicity**

Occurrence—Found in plants, all vertebrates

Specificity—Activity crosses species lines

Antigenicity—No antigenicity reported

2. **Units:** μg or mg; rabbit unit = 0.6 mg progesterone

3. **Normal Blood Levels**

Normal males—0.03 μg/100 ml plasma

Normal females—0.1-0.3 μg/100 ml plasma

Pregnant females—10-28 μg/100 ml plasma

4. **Administration**

Injection—Intramuscular

Topical—Not reported

Oral—As caproate or acetate of 17α-hydroxyprogesterone; various synthetic progestogens used in contraceptive pills in combination with small amounts of estrogens

5. **Factors Affecting Release**

Inhibitors

Psychic phenomena

Uterine factor
Feedback mechanisms via hypothalamus
Environmental factors
Stimulators
Hypothalamic agent—LRH (human)—via pituitary and LH
Males—Continuous secretion (low levels)
Females—Continuous secretion in nonspontaneous ovulators (rabbit, ferret, cat); rhythmic in spontaneous ovulators (dog, human)
Psychic and environmental controls
Prolactin or LH, depending on species

6. **Deficiency Symptoms (Humans)**
Termination of pregnancy
Decreased production of steroids
Decreased ovulation
Loss of normal cyclic changes
Decreased development for implantation and gestation

7. **Effects of Overdose, Excess**
Progestational changes
Pregnancy prolongation
Inhibition of uterine growth
Increased Na and K excretion

METABOLIC ROLE

1. **Biosynthesis:**   Acetate $\rightarrow$ Mevalonate $\rightarrow$ Squalene $\rightarrow$ Cholesterol $\rightarrow$ Pregnenolone $\rightarrow$ Progesterone
Cell Site: Microsomes

2. **Production Sites**
Ovary (follicles, corpus luteum)
Testicles (interstitial cells)
Adrenal cortex (reticularis fasciculata)
Placenta (syncytical trophoblast)

3. **Storage Sites**
Corpora lutea
Adrenal cortex

4. **Blood Carriers:**   Plasma lipoproteins—albumin, transcortin

5. **Half-life:**   About 5 min

6. **Target Tissues:**   Uterus, vagina, cervix, pubic symphysis, ovary, hypothalamus, mammary gland, female sex accessory organs, kidney, adrenal cortex, adenohypophysis

7. **Reactions:**   Reactive form—Unknown

Organ	Enzyme System	Effect
Uterus	Acid phosphatase	Activated
	Carbonic anhydrase	Activated

8. **Mode of Action**
   Cellular
      Anabolic: Increases glycoprotein (uterus). Increases glycogen (uterus)
      Catabolic: Increases protein catabolism. Increases galactose oxidation
      Other: Increases membrane potential. Immediate precursor for other
         sex hormones. Thermogenic action
   Organismal
      Increases kidney filtration rate (glomerulus)
      Promotes development and growth of uterus and mammary gland
      Promotes ovulation and development of sex accessories (female)
      Promotes excitation of uterus
      Inhibits release of LH

9. **Catabolism**
   Intermediates—Pregnanediol, 17α-hydroxyprogesterone
   Excretion products
      Urine—Mainly as glucuronates of pregnanediol, pregnanetriol
      Feces—Androgens (cow, rat)

MISCELLANEOUS

1. **Relationship to Vitamins**
   Niacin—DPN involved in progesterone synthesis
   Vitamin C—Depleted from adrenal cortex or ovary on progesterone
      formation

2. **Relationship to Other Hormones**
   Estradiol—Antagonist or synergist to progesterone, depending on concentration; made from progesterone

Prolactin, LH—Stimulant for production of progesterone, depending on species

Testosterone—Antagonist or synergist to progesterone, depending on concentration; made from progesterone

Cortisol, Aldosterone—Made from progesterone

STH, T4—Synergist in growth aspects of progesterone

ACTH—Releaser of steroids from adrenal cortex; stimulator of progesterone production

FSH—Synergist with LH in production of progesterone

Relaxin, Oxytocin—Synergist with progesterone in parturition

LRH—Hypothalamic agent stimulating release of LH

3. **Unusual Features**

Concentration dependence of effects

Primitive type of hormone

Causes maternal behavior in rabbit

Causes pseudopregnancy in nonspontaneous ovulators

Inhibits estrogenic tumors

Anesthetic effects

Androgenic or antiandrogenic, depending on species

Cyclic release in certain species but not in others

4. **Possible Relationships of Deficiency Symptoms to Metabolic Action**

Loss of pregnancy—Lack of growth and developmental stimulus to uterus by progesterone

Decreased steroid production—Serves as precursor to all other steroid hormones

Decreased ovulation—No progesterone stimulus for development of follicle in ovary

Loss of normal cyclic changes—Feedback mechanisms of progesterone on hypothalamus not controlling (?)

Decreased development for implantation and gestation—Loss of growth and development stimulating action on uterus due to lack of progesterone

35
Testosterone

GENERAL INFORMATION

1. Synonyms: 17β-Hydroxy-4-androsten-3-one, Δ^4-androsten-17β-ol-3-one

2. History

- 1849—Berthold demonstrated effects of castration prevented by testis transplants
- 1889—Brown-Sequard claimed rejuvenative powers of testicular extracts
- 1911—Pezard showed comb growth in capons by injection of testicular extracts
- 1927—McGee found extracts of bull testis highly potent for male sex hormone activity
- 1931—Butenandt isolated androsterone from human urine
- 1935—Laqueur crystallized testosterone from testicular extracts
- 1935—Butenandt, Ruzicka determined structure and synthesized testosterone

3. Physiological Forms: Androstenedione, testosterone, 11β-hydroxyandrostenedione, adrenosterone

4. Active Analogs and Related Compounds (Androgens)

Natural
- 11-Hydroxyandrosterone, adrenosterone, 7-hydroxyprogesterone
- 11-Keto-androsterone
- 11β-Hydroxyandrostenedione

Synthetic
Ethynyl testosterone, methyltestosterone
6α-chlorotestosterone,   19-nortestosterone,   17α-ethyl-19-nortesto-
sterone

5. Inactive Analogs and Related Compounds (for Androgenic Activity)
Cortisone, cortisol, 17-hydroxyprogesterone, lumiandrosterone
17α-hydroxy-11-desoxycorticosterone,   17β-methyl   epitestosterone,
etiocholanolone

6. Antagonists: Estrogens, (except in low concentrations), progesterone,
norethandrolone, 11α-hydroxyprogesterone, methylcholanthrene,
A-norprogesterone

7. Synergists: STH, insulin, other androgens, estrogens (in low concentrations)

8. Physiological Functions
Controls secondary male sex characteristics
Maintains functional competence of male reproductive ducts and glands
Increases protein anabolism; maintains spermatogenesis; inhibits gona-
dotrophin
Increases male sex behavior; increases closure of epiphyseal plates

9. Deficiency Diseases, Disorders
Male hypogonadism, eunuchoidism
Feminizing testes, hyperplasias of adrenals and testes

10. Essentiality for Life
Not essential for life of the organism, but essential for reproduction in all
(male) vertebrates

CHEMISTRY

1. Structure

Testosterone, $C_{19}H_{28}O_2$

2. **Reactions**

Heat—Stable

Acid—Esterifies

Alkali—Fluoresces (conc.)

Water—Insol.

Oxidation—Oxidizes to
androstenedione

Reduction—Unstable

Light—Stable

3. **Properties**

Appearance—White powder

MW—288.4

MP—155°C

Crystal Form—Needles

Salts, Esters

 Propionate, acetate,

 Butyrate, palmitate,

 Stearate, Benzoate

Important Groups for Activity

 $-C(3)=O,-C(17)-OH$

 $-C(4)=C(5)$

Solubility

 H_2O—Insol.

 Acet., Alc.—Sol.

 Benz., Chl., Eth.—Sol.

 Absn. Max.—238 mμ

Chemical Nature

 Alcoholic ketone, steroid

 $\alpha_D^{24} = 109°$

4. **Commercial Production**

Microbiological conversion of dehydroandrosterone

Synthesis from cholesterol

5. **Isolation**

Sources—Urine, blood

Method: Urine

 Hydrolyze with H_2SO_4, extract with organic solvents

 Precipitate with digitonin or Girard's reagent T

 Chromatography: $MgSiO_4$ column or paper or gas

Method: Blood

 Complex with methyl green; transesterify with acetic acid

 Chromatography on Florisil alumina columns

6. **Determination**

Bioassay

 Growth of capon comb

 Increase in various muscles

 Increase in weight of prostate

 Increase in fructose, citric acid in semen

 Maintenance of spermatogenesis in hypophysectomized rat

Physicochemical—Zimmerman   reaction-(17-oxosteroids);   Pettenkofer
 reaction

MEDICAL AND BIOLOGICAL ROLE

1. **Species Occurrence, Specificity, and Antigenicity**
   Occurrence—Vertebrates (cyclostomes and higher forms), variable types of androgens
   Specificity—Variable
   Mammals and Birds—testosterone and androsterone active; pregnenolone inactive
   Rat—pregnenolone active (not in mammals or birds)
   Antigenicity—None reported

2. **Units:** 0.015 mg = I.U.

3. **Normal Blood Levels (Man)**
   Males av. 0.60 μg/100 ml plasma—Androsterone and dehydroepiandrosterone; females av. 0.05 μg/100 ml plasma

4. **Administration**
   Injection—Intramuscular preferred
   Topical—Some cutaneous absorption
   Oral—Active, but less than injected or implanted hormones. More active as esters or synthetic androgens

5. **Factors Affecting Release**
   Inhibitors
      Cortisol
      Psychic effects
      Androgens
      Feedback to hypothalamus
   Stimulators
      Photoperiodicity
      Temperature increase, within limits
      Melatonin
      FSH, ACTH, LH, LRH
      Increased blood flow to testis
      Decreased blood levels of androgens or estrogens

6. **Deficiency Symptoms (Humans)**
   Involution of accessory organs (prostate, seminal vesicles)
   Decreased male behavior patterns and libido
   Decreased secondary sex traits
   Poor muscle development and function

Delayed closure of epiphyses
Decreased excretion of 17-keto-steroids in urine

7. **Effects of Overdose, Excess:** LD_{100} = 325 mg/kg in female rats
Increases libido
Virilization, acne
Increases fat catabolism
Increases androgen and estrogen excretion (17-keto-steroids)
Precocious sex development
Hypertrophy of accessory sex organs
Increases skeletal growth until epiphyses close
Increases muscle mass, hirsutism
Decreases scalp hair growth (?)
Decreases weight—chick, rat

METABOLIC ROLE

1. **Biosynthesis:**   Acetate → Mevalonate → Squalene → Cholesterol
→ Pregnenolone → Progesterone → 17α-hydroxyprogesterone
→ Androstenedione → Testosterone
Cell Sites: Leydig cells in interstitial cells of testis: Agranular cytoplasm

2. **Production Sites**
Interstitial cells of ovary and testis: Agranular cytoplasm
Adrenal cortex (reticularis fasciculata), embryonic placenta

3. **Storage Areas:**   No data

4. **Blood Carriers:**   Albumin, and a specific β-globulin

5. **Half-life:**   About 4 min

6. **Target Tissues**
Systemic, fat deposits, muscles, hypothalamus, kidney
Male sex organs, adenohypophysis, hair follicles
Epiphyses of long bones, vocal cords

7. **Reactions:**   Reactive forms
Redox couples—Testosterone ⇌ androstenedione ⇌ androsterone

Organ	Enzyme System	Effect
Kidney	β-Glucuronidase	Activated
	d-Aminooxidase	Activated
	Arginase	Activated
	Alkaline phosphatase	Inhibited
Prostate	Succinic dehydrogenase	Activated
Seminal vesicle	Amino acid activating enzymes	Activated

8. Mode of Action
Cellular

Anabolic—Increases incorporation of amino acids and protein synthesis in muscles, liver, kidney

Catabolic—Increases fat catabolism. Decreases amino acid catabolism

Other

Redox couple regulation of oxidation

Increased mitosis in certain tissues

Increases creatine storage

Membrane effects

Organismal

Increases development of male secondary sex organs and characteristics

Increases growth of muscles, liver, kidney

Androgenic, increases libido

Effects on CNS, male behavior

Increases folliculoid and luteoid activity in immature females

Increases basal metabolism

Maintains positive balances of N, K, Ca, P

Decreases creatinuria

Promotes closure of bone epiphyses

Stimulates red cell production

9. Catabolism
Intermediates—Androstanolone, androstanedione

Excretion Products—Androsterone, etiocholanolone, 17-keto-steroids, dehydroepiandrosterone. In urine, bile, feces-free or conjugated with sulfate or glucuronide. Enterohepatic circulation

MISCELLANEOUS

1. Relationship to Vitamins
Vitamins A, E, C, Folic Acid—Synergists with testosterone for maturation of germ cells and increased anabolic activity

Vitamin B Complex—Male accessory gland maintenance in rat (involution on vit. B deficiency, similar to castration); synergistic in increased metabolic rate

Vitamin D—Synergist with testosterone in bone metabolism

2. Relationship to Other Hormones

Estradiol—Formed from testosterone

LH, LRH, FSH—Stimulators of testosterone formation or release

Estradiol, STH, Insulin—Synergists for action of testosterone (in proper concentrations)

ACTH—stimulates formation of adrenal androgens

Progesterone, Estrogens—Antagonists to testosterone (in proper concentrations)

Cortisol, Estrogens, Androgens—Act as release inhibitors in high concentrations

3. Unusual Features

Multiple sources of production

Fetal sex determination to male via hypothalamus by testosterone

Sensitivity of capon comb to testosterone

Insensitivity of certain muscles to testosterone

Female birds produce testosterone in ovary

Immediate precursor in estrogen synthesis

Two major synthetic routes, three minor ones in adrenals and testes

Social functions in seals affected by androgens

Species differences in effects of testosterone on sperm maturation rate

Dietary effect—Vitamin B deficiency or protein deficiency similar to castration

4. Possible Relationships of Deficiency Symptoms to Metabolic Action

Involution of male accessory organs, decreased secondary sex traits—withdrawal of anabolic effect of testosterone

Decreased male behavior and libido—decreased effect on CNS

Poor muscle development and function—withdrawal of anabolic effect of testosterone

Delayed closure of epiphyses—withdrawal of anabolic effect of testosterone

Decreased excretion of 17-keto-steroids in urine—decreased production of androgens

36
Relaxin

GENERAL INFORMATION

1. **Synonyms:** Releasin, Cervilaxin

2. **History**
    1926—Hisaw cited evidence for a pregnancy hormone which causes relaxation of pelvic ligaments in preparation for parturition
    1930—Fevold *et al.* extracted relaxin from corpora lutea
    1942—Abramowitz isolated relaxin from pregnant rabbit serum
    1955—Lehrman *et al.* isolated and purified relaxin from ovaries of pregnant sows
    1966—Struck and Bhargava isolated first homogeneous preparations of relaxin

3. **Physiological Forms:** *l*-relaxin

4. **Active Analogs and Related Compounds:** Four similar peptides in relaxin family

5. **Inactive Analogs and Related Compounds:** Oxidized or reduced forms of relaxin

6. **Antagonists:** Androgens, corticosterone, high levels of estradiol and progesterone

7. **Synergists:** Low levels of estradiol and progesterone, oxytocin, T4

8. **Physiological Functions**
     Enlargement of birth canal in preparation for parturition
     Separation of symphysis pubis, loss of rigidity in pelvic bones
     Decreases uterine motility
     Maintenance of pregnancy (progesterone + estrogen sparing)
     Increases sensitivity to oxytocin
     Releases oxytocin
     Stimulates mammary gland
     Stimulates imbibition of water in uterus
     Inhibits uterine contraction

9. **Deficiency Diseases, Disorders:**   None known

10. **Essentiality for Life:**   Not essential for human female reproduction, but is essential for other mammalian reproduction. Otherwise not essential for life

CHEMISTRY

1. **Structure:**   Polypeptide (4 peptides with activity have been isolated). Contains Ala, Asp, Cys, Glu, Gly, His, Lys, Ser, Tyr, Val, Arg, guanidine. About 30-40 amino acids in each peptide

2. **Reactions**

    Heat—Stable to 100°C neut. soln.

    Acid—Inactivates (in acidic methanol)

    Alkali—Inactivates (in hot alkali)

    Water—Sol. (acidic)

    Oxidation—Inactivates

    Reduction—Inactivates (SH agents)

    Light—No data

    Proteolytic enzymes—Inactivate

3. **Properties**

    Appearance—Amorphous powder

    MW—4000-5000

    MP—No data

    Crystal Form—Amorphous

    Salts—No data

    Important Groups for Activity
      Guanidine   S—S
              Cys

    Solubility
      H_2O—Sl. sol.
      Acet., Alc.—Insol.
      Benz., Chl., Eth.—Insol.
    Absn. Max.—277.5 mμ
    Chemical Activity—Acidic polypeptide
    Misc.—pl = 4.4

4. **Commercial Production**
   Isolation from pregnant sow ovaries

5. **Isolation**
   Source—Pregnant sow ovaries
   Method—Extraction with trichloroacetic acid, glacial acetic acid, acid-
      acetone; chromatography on columns of DEAE cellulose, IRC-50;
      gel filtration on sephadex G-50

6. **Determination of potency and concentration**
   Bioassay—Measure length of interpubic ligament in mice
      X-Ray photography of innominate bones in estrogen primed guinea
      pig
   Inhibition of motility of mouse uterine segments in vitro
   Physico-chemical—None

MEDICAL AND BIOLOGICAL ROLE

1. **Species Occurrence, Specificity, and Antigenicity**
   Occurrence—Found in mammals, birds, sharks. Relaxin-like substances
      have been isolated from elasmobranch ovaries and bird testes
   Specificity—High; species differences pronounced
   Antigenicity—Moderate; can be antigenic

2. **Units:** Guinea pig units. Minimal amount necessary to cause appreciable
   separation of symphysis in guinea pig

3. **Normal Blood Levels:** 200 GPU/100 ml (pregnant sow)

4. **Administration**
   Injection—Usually used
   Topical—Not active
   Oral—Not active

5. **Factors Affecting Release**
   Inhibitors
      Androgens
      Corticosterone
      High progesterone level
      High estradiol level

Stimulators
    Low estradiol level
    Low progesterone level
    Pregnenolone

6. **Deficiency Symptoms:**   Humans—Unknown

7. **Effects of Overdose, Excess:**   Unknown.

METABOLIC ROLE

1. **Biosynthesis**
    Precursors
        11 of 20 standard amino acids, progesterone (cofactor)
        Reducing sugars
        Missing: Try, Asn, Gln, Met, Leu, Ile, Phe, Thr, Pro
    Intermediates—Unknown
    Site(s) in Cell—Unknown

2. **Production Sites:**   Corpus luteum in pregnancy. Possibly placenta, uterus in some species

3. **Storage Areas:**   None

4. **Blood Carriers:**   Unknown

5. **Half-life:**   Approx. 1 hr

6. **Target Tissues**
    Connective tissue of pubic symphysis
    Uterus (diminution of contractions and softening of cervix)
    Mammary gland
    Vagina

7. **Reactions:**   Reactive Forms: Unknown

Organ	Enzyme System	Effect
Pubic symphysis	Collagen depolymerases	Activated
Liver	Cholesterol biosynthesis	Inhibited
Uterus	Alkaline phosphatase	Increased

8. Mode of Action
Cellular
  Anabolic—Increases uterine glycogen synthesis
  Catabolic—No data
Other—Decreases membrane potential of myometrium. Enzyme activator
Organismal
  Increases vascularity of pubic symphysis
  Imbibition of water; disaggregation and depolymerization of muco-
    proteins in ground structure of symphysis
  Increases glycogen and water content of uterus, also dry weight and
    N content
  Decreases uterine motility
  Softens cervix of uterus
  Increases uterine sensitivity to oxytocin
  Stimulates release of oxytocin
  Relaxes interpubic ligament

9. Catabolism
Intermediates—Peptides, amino acids
Excretion products—Ammonia, CO_2, H_2O, amino acids, 1-4% relaxin in
  urine

MISCELLANEOUS

1. **Relationship to Vitamins:** Vitamin C—Maintains mucoprotein ground
   substance in connective tissue, affected by relaxin

2. **Relationship to Other Hormones**
   Estradiol—Relaxin works in conjunction with estrogens—synergistic or
     antagonistic depending on concentration (requires estrogen
     "priming")
   Oxytocin—Relaxin may initiate oxytocin release
   STH—Relaxin may require growth hormone for relaxation of interpubic
     ligament
   Progesterone—Synergistic or antagonistic depending on concentration
   TSH—Increased biosynthesis of TSH stimulated by relaxin
   Testosterone, Corticosterone—Act as release inhibitors

3. **Unusual Features**
   Hormone of pregnancy only
   Strictly female hormone, although general effects noted in body

Found in rooster testes—No known function
Inhibits cholesterol biosynthesis, hypocholesteremic
Increases hydrolysis of collagen

4. Possible Relationships of Deficiency Symptoms to Metabolic Action:
Unknown

37
Epinephrine

GENERAL INFORMATION

1. **Synonyms:** Adrenaline, Adrenin, Suprarenin, Vasotonin, Vasocon-
   strictine, Adrenamine, Levorenine

2. **History**
   1895—Oliver and Shafer demonstrated pressor effect of suprarenal
      extracts
   1899—Abel named pressor agent epinephrine
   1901—Takamine, Aldrich isolated epinephrine from animal adrenal
      glands
   1904—Stolz ⎱
   1905—Dakin ⎰ synthesized *dl*-epinephrine
   1908—Flacher responsible for resolution of *dl*-form of epinephrine
   1910—Barger and Dale defined sympathomimetic amines and their
      properties
   1958—Pratesi determined configuration of epinephrine

3. **Physiological Forms:** *l*-Epinephrine

4. **Active Analogs and Related Compounds**
   d-epinephrine (1/15 as active as *l*-isomers), norepinephrine, dopamine,
      ephedrin, benzedrine, paredrine, tyramine, isoproterenol

5. **Inactive Analogs and Related Compounds:** DOPA

6. **Antagonists:**   Insulin, ergotamine, dibenamine, oxytocin, dibenzyline, tetraethylammonium chloride

7. **Synergists:**   Glucagon, T4, cortisol, ACTH

8. **Physiological Functions**

Blood Circulation—Increases blood pressure (pressor agent), peripheral vasodilator, increases heart output and rate, flow increase in brain, liver, and skeletal muscle

Kidney—Reduces glomerular filtration rate

Lung, intestine, genital system—Inhibited motility

Metabolic effects—Increases O_2 consumption, increases temperature, increases BMR, increases gluconeogenesis

CNS effects—Restlessness, anxiety

Pituitary effects—Stimulates production and release of ACTH and corticoids

Emergency hormone—Stress reactions

9. **Deficiency Diseases, Disorders:**   Pheochromocytoma (chromaffin cells)

10. **Essentiality for Life:**   Not absolutely essential for life of organism; possible shortening of life span due to decreased response to emergencies

CHEMISTRY

1. **Structure**

l-Epinephrine, $C_9H_{13}NO_3$

2. **Reactions**

Heat—Decomposes at $215°C$

Acid—Inactivates

Alkali—Unstable—Very sol. in dil. NaOH. Insol. in NH_4OH

Water—Sol., basic

Oxidation—Oxidizes easily

Reduction—Stable

Light—Fluorescent in UV; darkens on exposure, forms adrenochrome

3. **Properties**

Appearance—white crystalline powder

MW—183.2

MP—211-212°C

Crystal Form—No data

Salts—HCl

Important Groups for Activity

Phenol, amine, alcohol

$-C(4)OH, -NH-, -CHOH$

Solubility

H_2O—Sparingly

Acet., Alc.—Insol.

Benz., Chl., Eth.—Insol.

Absn. Max.—279 mμ

Chemical Nature

Catecholamine

Secondary amine

$\alpha_D^{25} = -53.5°$ (0.5 N HCl)

4. **Commercial Production**

Adrenal gland extractions

Synthetic production

5. **Isolation**

Sources—Adrenal medulla, urine, blood

Methods

Hydrolysis of conjugates, if any, boiling at pH 2, 20 min

Extraction with acidic ethanol or n-butanol

Purification via paper chromatography

6. **Determination**

Bioassay

Inhibition of movement of isolated rat uterus

Constrictor action on artery of denervated rabbit ear

Physicochemical

Iodochrome oxidation to distinguish norepinephrine from epinephrine

Fluorescence in alkali

Color reaction with ferric chloride

MEDICAL AND BIOLOGICAL ROLE

1. **Species Occurrence, Specificity, and Antigenicity**

Occurrence—Found in all vertebrates and some invertebrates

Specificity—None, full interspecific potency

Antigenicity—None

2. **Units:**   None; by weight

3. **Normal Blood Levels (Man):**   Approximately 0.01 μg/100 ml plasma (venous)

4. **Administration**
    Injection—Subcutaneous, intramuscular
    Topical—Active (electrophoretic application)
    Oral—Possible, but slow

5. **Factors Affecting Release**
    Inhibitors—Nerve controls, excess catecholamines
    Stimulators—Nicotine, histamine, reserpine, acetylcholine, morphine,
        ether, ACTH, glucocorticoids, low blood sugar, stress, insulin,
        psychic (hypothalamus) nerve controls, trauma, exercise

6. **Deficiency Symptoms** Not fatal, but organism cannot respond to emer-
    gency, hard work, temperature extreme, emotional disturbance

7. **Effects of Overdose, Excess**
    Decreases oxygen consumption, BMR, clotting time,
    Tachycardia, restlessness, anxiety, fatigue, inhibited G.I. tract,
    Increases heart rate, respiration, pallor, blood sugar, sweat, blood flow
        (muscle)
    Ventricular fibrillation, paroxystic or sustained hypertension

METABOLIC ROLE

1. **Biosynthesis:**   Phenylalanine → Tyrosine → 3,4-Dihydroxyphenylalanine
    (DOPA) → 3,4-Dihydroxyphenylethylamine (Dopamine) → Nore-
    pinephrine → Epinephrine
    Site(s) in cell: In golgi (osmiophilic granules)

2. **Production Sites:**   Chromaffin cells in gut and adrenal medulla

3. **Storage Areas:**   Chromaffin cells in liver and gut

4. **Blood Carriers:**   Free in blood or conjugated with sulfate or glucuronides,
    or combined with albumin

5. **Half-life:**   About 2 min

6. **Target Tissues:**   Systemic, vascular system, liver, muscles

7. **Reactions**
    Reactive intermediate—Cyclic AMP—(secondary messenger)

Organ	Enzyme System	Effect
Muscle and liver	Phosphorylase b	Activated
	Adenyl cyclase	Activated
	Phosphorylase b kinase	Activated
	Synthetase I kinase	Activated
	Synthetase I	Inhibited
Adipose tissue	Lipase	Activated
	Adenyl cyclase	Activated

8. Mode of Action
Cellular

Anabolic—No data

Catabolic —Increases glycogenolysis in liver, increases fat catabolism

Other

Decreases glucose entry into cells of skeletal muscle

Increases glucose entry into heart, brain and adipose tissue cells

Increases cyclic AMP

Supresses mitosis

Calorigenic action

Organismal

Increases—Systolic pressure; blood flow to skeletal muscles, liver; blood sugar; lipolysis; blood K^+; O_2 consumption (BMR), glucose absorption from gut, mental alertness, sweating

Decreases—Glucose tolerance, eosinophils, blood flow to capillaries of skin and kidney, plasma volume

Lightens chromatophores

9. Catabolism
Intermediates—3,4-dihydroxymandelic acid

Excretion Products—Free (0.5 to 2%) or as metanephrine (3-methoxy, 4OH-mandelic acid)

MISCELLANEOUS

1. **Relationship to Vitamins:**   Vitamin C—Maintains reduced state of epinephrine. Vitamins C, B_6, B_{12}, folic acid—Cofactors in synthesis of epinephrine from phenylalanine

2. **Relationship to Other Hormones**

Norepinephrine—Immediate precursor to epinephrine

Insulin—Antagonist to epinephrine

Glucagon, T4, ACH—Synergists to epinephrine

TSH—Released by epinephrine
Prolactin—Blocking of milk ejection by epinephrine
Cortisol, Cortisone—Synergistic in stress response
Oxytocin—Epinephrine antagonistic in milk ejection

3. Unusual Features

Active at 1.4 parts per billion
Absent in developing fetus; Proportion of NOR/EP = 1:4 in adult human
    adrenal (reverse in chick); blocks milk ejection; rabbit most
    sensitive; behavioral effects
Proportion of NOR/EP varies in invertebrates
Increases mental alertness
Calorigenic action

4. Possible Relationships of Deficiency Symptoms to Metabolic Action

Decreased emergency response—Decreased lipolysis in adipose tissue
    results in decreased glucose energy (ATP) available for stress
    reaction
Decreased response to emotional disturbances, temperature extremes,
    hard work—as in the previous symptom

38
Norepinephrine

GENERAL INFORMATION

1. **Synonyms:** Noradrenaline, arterenol, levarterenol

2. **History**

   1898—Lewandowsky ⎫ Noted similarity of effects of adrenal gland
   1901—Langley ⎭ extracts and stimulation of sympathetic nerves, on tissues

   1904—Eliot proposed sympathetic nerve endings release epinephrine-like substance

   1910—Barger and Dale synthesized norepinephrine

   1927—Cannon and Uridil noted that liver releases epinephrine-like substance called sympathin on stimulation of sympathetic nerves

   1948—Tullar resolved *dl*-form of norepinephrine

   1951—Euler demonstrated sympathin to be norepinephrine

   1959—Pratesi established configuration of norepinephrine

3. **Physiological Forms:** *l*-Norepinephrine

4. **Active Analogs and Related Compounds:** Dopamine, ephedrine, *d*-norepinephrine, *d*-epinephrine (1/15 as active as *l*-isomers)

5. **Inactive Analogs and Related Compounds:** DOPA

6. **Antagonists:** Insulin, vasopressin

7. **Synergists:**   Epinephrine, serotonin, cortisol, cortisone, glucagon

8. **Physiological Functions**
    Blood circulation—Increases blood pressure, peripheral vasoconstrictor, without change or slight decrease in output and heart rate. No flow increase in brain, liver, or muscle
    Kidney—Decreases glomerular filtration rate
    Lung, intestine, genital system—Inhibited
    Metabolic effects—Weak epinephrine effect.
    CNS effects—Adrenergic transmitter agent at synapses, no brain excitation
    Pituitary effects—None
    Maintenance hormone—Diurnal regulation
    Immediate precursor of epinephrine

9. **Deficiency Diseases, Disorders**
    Neuroblastoma
    Pheochromocytoma

10. **Essentiality for Life:**   Not absolutely essential for life of organism, except if other neurotransmitters not available

CHEMISTRY

1. **Structure**

l-Norepinephrine, $C_8H_{11}NO_3$

2. **Reactions**

Heat—Unstable	Oxidation—Easily oxidizes to
Acid—Inactivates	noradrenochrome
Alkali—Very sol. dil. NaOH;	Reduction—Stable
Insol. NH_4OH	Light—No fluorescence in UV
Water—Soluble, alkaline	

3. **Properties**

Appearance—Colorless crystals	Salts—HCl
MW—169.2	Important Groups for Activity
MP—145-146°C	Alcohol—CHOH, phenol,
Crystal Form—No data	—C(4)OH, amine, (—NH_2)

Solubility

  H_2O sparingly

  Acet., Alc.—Sl. sol.

  Benz., Chl., Eth.—Sl. sol.

  Absn. Max.—279 mμ

Chemical Nature—Catecholamine;

  primary amine

$\alpha_D^{25} = -37.3$ (HCl)

Misc.—pK = 8.8, 9.98

4. **Commercial Production:** Synthetic production

5. **Isolation**

  Sources—Adrenal medulla, blood, urine

  Methods

    Hydrolysis of conjugates, if any—Boil at pH 2, 20 min

    Extraction with acidic ethanol or *n*-butanol

6. **Determination**

  Bioassay—Pressor effect in cat, rat

  Physicochemical

    Colorimetric—Ferric chloride complex

    Fluorometric—Condense with ethylenediamine

MEDICAL AND BIOLOGICAL ROLE

1. **Species, Occurrence, Specificity, and Antigenicity**

  Occurrence—Found in all vertebrates and some invertebrates

  Specificity—None; full, interspecific potency

  Antigenicity—None

2. **Units:** None; by weight

3. **Normal Blood Levels (Man):** Approx. 0.05 μg/100 ml plasma (venous)

4. **Administration**

  Injection—Usual

  Topical—By electrophoresis through skin

  Oral—Inactive

5. **Factors Affecting Release**

  Inhibitors—Nerve controls, excess catecholamines

  Stimulators—ACH, nicotine, histamine, Tyr, Phe, low blood sugar, low
    T4, nerve controls, stress, trauma, reserpine, morphine

6. **Deficiency Symptoms**

 Poor nerve condition

 Orthostatic hypotension—Fainting on standing up, dizziness, light-headedness

7. **Effects of Overdose, Excess:** Bradycardia, pheochromocytoma

METABOLIC ROLE

1. **Biosynthesis:** Phenylalanine → Tyrosine → 3,4-Dihydroxyphenylalanine (DOPA) → 3,4-Dihydroxyphenylethylamine (Dopamine) — Norepinephrine

 Site(s) in cell—Osmiophilic granules in golgi apparatus

2. **Production Sites**

 Adrenal medulla

 Adrenergic nerve endings

 Chromaffin cells—sympathetic nerves and ganglia, gut

3. **Storage Areas:** Chromaffin cells in liver and gut, intraaxonal spaces, adrenal medulla

4. **Blood Carriers:** Free or sulfate, glucuronide esters

5. **Half-life:** 2 min or less

6. **Target Tissues:** Systemic, esp. vascular system, lung, eye

7. **Reactions:** Reactive intermediate: Cyclic AMP—secondary messenger

Organ	Enzyme Systems	Effect
Muscle and liver	Adenyl cyclase	Activated
	Phosphorylase b	Activated
	Phosphorylase b kinase	Activated
	Synthetase I kinase	Activated
	Synthetase I	Inhibited
Adipose tissue	Adenyl cyclase	Activated
	Lipase	Activated

8. **Mode of Action**

 Cellular

 Anabolic—No data

Catabolic
Increased CHO catabolism
Increased glycogen to glucose conversion
Increased fat catabolism
Other—No data
Organismal
Decreases—Pulse, blood flow, G.I. and genital activity, respiration
Increases—Diastolic and systolic pressure, vasodilation of coronary arteries, lipid mobilization, glucose absorption from gut
Bradycardia
Vasoconstrictor

9. **Catabolism**
Intermediates—3,4-dihydroxymandelic acid
Excretion products—Free in urine (3-6%), normetanephrine, 3-methoxy, 4-hydroxymandelic acid

MISCELLANEOUS

1. **Relationship to Vitamins:**   Vitamin C protects against oxidation of norepinephrine. Vitamins B_6, C, folic acid—cofactors in synthesis of norepinephrine from phenylalanine

2. **Relationship to Other Hormones**
Epinephrine—Derivative of norepinephrine; synergist also
Insulin—Antagonist to norepinephrine, secretion inhibited by norepinephrine
Serotonin, Cortisol, Cortisone—Synergists to norepinephrine
T4, ACH—Stimulators for release of norepinephrine

3. **Unusual Features**
Neurohumor—Much carried intraaxonally
EP/NOR = 4/1 in medulla (man)
Diurnal (higher in day)
No behavioral effects
Increases pigment concentration in skin
Main amine in fetus
Anticipatory type, i.e., normal plasma maintenance

4. **Possible Relationships of Deficiency Symptoms to Metabolic Action**
Poor nerve conduction—Lack of transmitter agent
Dizziness, light-headedness, fainting—Low blood pressure

Summarizing
Tables

TABLE 1. Characteristics of Vitamins

(+ = present in structure or function ± = slightly)
(— = catabolic or inhibiting effect)

Structural Component or Function	A	B_1	B_2	B_6	B_{12}	C	D	E	K	Biotin	F.A.[a]	Niacin	P.A.[b]
Amino Acid										+	+		+
Purine, pyrimidine (derivative)		+	+		+						+		
Benzene ring			+					+			+		
Pyridine ring				+								+	
Isoprene group (derivative)	+						+	+	+				
Sugar (derivative)			+		+	+							
Alcohol groups	+	+	+	+	+	+	+	+			+		+
Double bonds (—C=C—)	+	+	+	+	+	+	+	+	+		+	+	
Elements other than CHON		S			Co					S			
Redox agent			+			+	+	+	+		+	+	
PO_4 complex *in vivo*		+	+	+	+	+	+				+	+	+
Antioxidant			+		+	+		+					
Biosynthesis via Cholesterol pathway	+						+		+				

Anabolic functions	+	+	+	+	+	+	+	+	+	+	+	+
Catabolic functions	+	+	±	+	+	+	+	+	+	+	+	+
Stored in organism (man)	±	±	±	±	±	±	±	±	+	±	+	±
Available from intestinal bacteria (man)	±	±					±	+	+			
Toxic in excess (man)	+	+	+	+	+	±	+		+		+	
Mitosis effect		+	+	−				+				
Mitochondrial sites	+	+	+	+	+	+	+	+		+		
Chloroplast sites	+[g]	+					+	+		+		
Microsomal sites				+	+	+			+			
Membrane sites	+	+	+	+	+	+	+					
Protein synthesis				+	±	+						
Amino acid synthesis		−	−	+	±	+			±		−	−
CHO synthesis	+	−	−	+	+	+	+		+		−	−

[a]Folic acid. [b]Pantothenic acid. [g]Carotenoids.

TABLE 1. Characteristics of Vitamins (cont.)

(+ = stimulating effect or present in organelles)

Structural Component or Function	A	B_1	B_2	B_6	B_{12}	C	D	E	K	Biotin	F.A.[a]	Niacin	P.A.[b]
TCA Cycle effect		+	+									+	+
Lipid synthesis					+							±	±
Fatty acid synthesis				+						+			±
Nucleic acid synthesis					+								
Purine pyrimidine synthesis					+					+	+		
Mineral metabolism	Ca					Fe, Ca	Ca	Se					
H$_2$O metabolism													+
Hormone Synthesis	Prog.[e] ACH[f] Cortic.[c] Andro.[d]	ACH[f]		Nor. Serot.		Serot. Gluc.						+	ACH[f]
Sterol Synthesis	+			+		+						+	+

[a]Folic acid. [b]Pantothenic acid. [c]Corticosterone. [d]Androstenedione. [e]Progesterone. [f]Acetylcholine.

TABLE 2. Synergisms (+) and Antagonisms (−) Among the Vitamins

Vitamins	A	B_1	B_2	B_6	B_{12}	C	D	E	K	Biotin	F.A.[a]	Niacin	P.A.[b]
A			+	+	+	±							
B_1			+	+	+							+	+
B_2	+	+		+	+				+	+		+	+
B_6		+	+			+	+	+	+	+			
B_{12}	+	+	+			+	+	+	+	+		+	+
C	+		+	+			+	+		+			+
D												+	
E			+	+	+		+			+			
K						+	+						
Biotin			+	+	+						+		+
F.A.[a]			+	+	+	+	+	+		+		+	+
Niacin		+	+	+	+		+			+			+
P.A.[b]		+	+	+	+			+			+	+	

[a] Folic acid. [b] Pantothenic acid.

TABLE 3. Characteristics of Hormones

Hormones[a]	Amino Acid Units (Proteins, Peptides)	S—S Bonds	CHO Component	Steroid Unit	Catecholamine	Elements Other Than CHON	Redox Couple in Vivo	Mediated Via Cyclic AMP	CHO Anabolism + / Catabolism −	Lipid or Fat Anabolism + / Catabolism −	Protein (Amino Acid) Anabolism + / Catabolism −	Nucleic Acid (or Purine, pyrim.) Anabolism + / Catabolism −	Steroid Anabolism + / Catabolism −	Mineral and H₂O Balance	Mitotic Effect (Increase +, Decrease −)	Membrane Effect	Kidney Function	Blood Pressure	Nerve Function
ACTH	+					S		+	−	−			+[b]						
Aldos.				+			+		±	−	±	±		+		+	+		
Cort.				+			+		±	±	±	±		+	−	+	+		
Epi.					+		+	+	−	±			+[b]	+	−	+	+	+	+
Est.				+					±	+	+	+	+	+	+	+			+
FSH	+	+	+			S		+	+		+		+			+			
Gluc.	+					S		+	−	−	−			+		+	+		
GH (STH)	+	+				S		+	+	−	+	+		+	+	+	+		
(HRH)	+	+				S		+								+			

In.	+	+	S	+	±	+	+	+	+	+	+	
LH	+	+	S	+	–	+	+	+	+	+		
MSH	+		S	+			+		+			
Norepi.		+		+	–	–			+	+	+	+
Oxy.	+	+	S	+				+	+	+		
PTH	+		S	+	–		+	+	+	+		
Prog.				±	±	±	+	+	+	+	+	+
Prol.	+	+	S	+	+	–	+	+	+	+	+	+
Relax.	+	+	S	+	±	±	+	+	+			
Test.			+	–	–		+	+	+	+	+	+
TCT	+	+	S	+	+	+	+	+	+	+	+	
T4	+		I	+	–	–	+	+	+	+	+	+
TSH	+	+	S	+	±	–	+	+		+		
Vaso.	+	+	S	+	–		+	+	+	+	+	+

aSee list of abbreviations for full name. bRelease.

TABLE 4. Synergisms (+) and Antagonisms (−)

Hormones[a]	ACTH	Aldos.	Cort.	Epi.	Est.	FSH.	Gluc.	GH (STH)	HRH	In.	LH
ACTH			±	+				±		−	
Aldos.			−		−			+			
Cort.	±	−		+	±	+		±		−	
Epi.	+		+				+			−	
Est.		−	±					+		+	
FSH								+			+
Gluc.			+	+						−	
GH (STH)	±	+	±		+	+				±	
HRH											
In.	−		−	−	+	−	−	±			±
LH				+						±	
MSH			±	−				+			
Norepi.			+	+			+			−	
Oxy.		+	±	−	+			+			
PTH			±		±[b]			−			
Prog.		−	+		±			+			
Prol.			+		±			+			±
Relax.			−		±						
Test.			−		±			+		+	
TCT					+						
T4	±		+	+	+	+		+		−	+
TSH	+							+			
Vaso.		±	−	+				+			

[a] See list of abbreviations for full name.   [b] Birds.

Among the Hormones

Hormones[a]	MSH	Norepi.	Oxy.	PTH	Prog.	Prol.	Relax.	Test.	TCT	T4	TSH	Vaso.
ACTH										±	+	
Aldos.			+	−								±
Cort.	±	+	±	±	+	+	−	−		+		−
Epi.	−	+	−							+		+
Est.			+	±[b]	±	±	±	±	+	+		
FSH										+		
Gluc.		+										
GH (STH)	+		+	−	+	+		+		+	+	+
HRH												
In.		−						+		−		
LH					±					+		
MSH										+	+	
Norepi.												−
Oxy.				±	+	+				+		
PTH					+			−	−	−		
Prog.			±			+	±	±		+		
Prol.			+	+	+			−		+		+
Relax.			+		±			−		+		
Test.				−	±	−	−					+
TCT				−								
T4	+		+	−	+	+	+				+	+
TSH	+									+		
Vaso.		−				+		+		+		

[a]See list of abbreviations for full name.   [b]Birds.

TABLE 5. Synergisms (+) and Antagonisms (−) Between Vitamins and Hormones

Hormones[a]	A	B₁	B₂	B₆	B₁₂	C	D	E	K	Biotin	F.A.[b]	Niacin	P.A.[c]
ACTH	+									+		+	+
Aldos.													
Cort.						±	−						
Epi.				+		+							
Est.	−		−				+	+			+		
FSH													
Gluc.				+									
GH (STH)	+	+	+	+	+	+	+	+	+	+	+	+	+
					All related to growth								
HRH													
In.		+	+		−								
LH							+						
MSH	+												
Norepi.				+		+							
Oxy.													
PTH							±						
Prog.													
Prol.[e]	+	+	+	+	+·	+	+	+	+	+	+	+	±
Relax.													
Test.	+	+	+			+	+	+		+	+		
TCT						−							
T4	±[d]	+	+	−		+		−				+	
TSH	−[d]		+										
Vaso.													

[a] See list of abbreviations for full name. [b] Folic acid. [c] Pantothenic acid. [d] Large Doses.
[e] All synergistic when acting as a growth hormone.

TABLE 6. Principal Functional Relationships of Vitamins and Hormones

( ) = indirect effect ____= Major Effect

Function	Vitamin(s)[a]	Hormone(s)[a]
Bone and Ca metabolism	A, C, <u>D</u>	Cort., (ACTH), Est., GH <u>PTH</u>, Test., <u>TCT</u>, T4, (TSH)
Circulation, blood cells	B_6, B_{12}, C, E, K, Bio., <u>F.A.</u>, P.A.	Cort., (ACTH), <u>Epi.</u>, Norepi., Vaso.
Digestion and absorption	B_1, B_{12}, <u>D</u>, <u>E</u>, F.A., <u>Nia.</u>	Cort., (ACTH), Gluc., <u>In.</u>, PTH, <u>T4</u> (TSH)
Epithelium, skin (membrane effect)	<u>A</u>, B_2, B_{12}, D, <u>Bio.</u>, P.A.	Aldos., Cort., (ACTH), Epi., Est., GH, In., Norepi., Oxy., Prog., Relax., Test., T4 (TSH), <u>Vaso.</u>
Fat and CHO metabolism	<u>B_1</u>, <u>B_2</u>, B_6, B_{12}, Bio., Nia., <u>P.A.</u>	(ACTH), Aldos., Cort., Epi., Est., <u>Gluc.</u>, GH, <u>In.</u>, Norepi., T4 (TSH), Test.
Growth	All, by definition	All, by definition; Esp.: <u>Est.</u>, <u>GH</u>, <u>In.</u>, <u>T4</u> (TSH), <u>Test.</u>
Metabolic rate, temperature (TCA Cycle)	<u>B_1</u>, <u>B_2</u>, C, E, K, <u>Nia.</u>, P.A.	Epi., Norepi., Prog., <u>T4</u>, (TSH), Test.
Nerve function, psyche	A, <u>B_1</u>, B_2, B_{12}, C, Bio., Nia., <u>F.A.</u>, P.A.	Cort., (ACTH), <u>Epi.</u>, Norepi., Prol., Test., <u>T4</u>, (TSH), Est.
Pigmentation	B_6, C, F.A., <u>Nia.</u>	(ACTH), Cort., <u>MSH</u>
Pregnancy, lactation	All required at higher levels	Cort., (ACTH), <u>Est.</u> (FSH), GH, In., (LH), <u>Oxy.</u>, <u>Prol.</u>, <u>Prog.</u>, <u>Relax.</u>, T4, (TSH)
Salt (Na) and H_2O metabolism	B_6, <u>P.A.</u> (A, C, E, Nia.)	<u>Aldos.</u>, Cort., (ACTH), Epi., Gluc., GH, (In.), Norepi., Oxy., Prog., T4, (TSH), <u>Vaso.</u>
Stress, immunity	<u>C</u>, P.A., <u>A</u> (B_1, B_2, B_6, K, Bio., F.A.)	Aldo., <u>Cort.</u>, (ACTH), Est.
Visual mechanisms	<u>A</u>, B_2	

[a] See list of abbreviations for full name.

TABLE 7. Food and Nutrition Board, National Academy of Science— National Research Council Recommended Daily Dietary Allowances,[1] Revised 1968

Designed for the maintenance of good nutrition of practically all healthy people in the U.S.A.

	Age[2] Years From Up to	Weight Kg (lb)		Height cm (in.)		Kcal	Protein g	Vit. A Activity I.U.	Vit. D I.U.	Vit. E Activity I.U.
								Fat Soluble Vitamins		
Infants	0–1/6	4	9	55	22	kg x 120	kg x 2.2[5]	1500	400	5
	1/6–1/2	7	15	63	25	kg x 110	kg x 2.0[5]	1500	400	5
	1/2–1	9	20	72	28	kg x 100	kg x 1.8[5]	1500	400	5
Children	1–2	12	26	81	32	1100	25	2000	400	10
	2–3	14	31	91	36	1250	25	2000	400	10
	3–4	16	35	100	39	1400	30	2500	400	10
	4–6	19	42	110	43	1600	30	2500	400	10
	6–8	23	51	121	48	2000	35	3500	400	15
	8–10	28	62	131	52	2200	40	3500	400	15
Males	10–12	35	77	140	55	2500	45	4500	400	20
	12–14	43	95	151	59	2700	50	5000	400	20
	14–18	59	130	170	67	3000	60	5000	400	25
	18–22	67	147	175	69	2800	60	5000	400	30
	22–35	70	154	175	69	2800	65	5000	–	30
	35–55	70	154	173	68	2600	65	5000	–	30
	55–75+	70	154	171	67	2400	65	5000	–	30
Females	10–12	35	77	142	56	2250	50	4500	400	20
	12–14	44	97	154	61	2300	50	5000	400	20
	14–16	52	114	157	62	2400	55	5000	400	25
	16–18	54	119	160	63	2300	55	5000	400	25
	18–22	58	128	163	64	2000	55	5000	400	25
	22–35	58	128	163	64	2000	55	5000	–	25
	35–55	58	128	160	63	1850	55	5000	–	25
	55–75+	58	128	157	62	1700	55	5000	–	25
Pregnancy						+200	65	6000	400	30
Lactation						+1000	75	8000	400	30

1. The allowance levels are intended to cover individual variations among most normal persons as they live in the United States under usual environmental stresses. The recommended allowances can be attained with a variety of common foods, providing other nutrients for which human requirements have been less well defined. See text [of Recommended Dietary Allowances, National Research Council Pub. # 1694] for more detailed discussion of allowances and of nutrients not tabulated.

2. Entries on lines for age range 22–35 years represent the reference man and woman at age 22. All other entries represent allowances for the midpoint of the specified age range.

	Water Soluble Vitamins						Minerals				
Ascorbic Acid mg	Folacin[3] mg	Niacin mg. equiv.[4]	Ribo-flavin mg	Thiamine mg	Vit. B_6 mg	Vit. B_{12} µg	Calcium gm	Phos-phorus gm	Iodine µg	Iron mg	Mag-nesium mg
35	0.05	5	0.4	0.2	0.2	1.0	0.4	0.2	25	6	40
35	0.05	7	0.5	0.4	0.3	1.5	0.5	0.4	40	10	60
35	0.1	8	0.6	0.5	0.4	2.0	0.6	0.5	45	15	70
40	0.1	8	0.6	0.6	0.5	2.0	0.7	0.7	55	15	100
40	0.2	8	0.7	0.6	0.6	2.5	0.8	0.8	60	15	150
40	0.2	9	0.8	0.7	0.7	3	0.8	0.8	70	10	200
40	0.2	11	0.9	0.8	0.9	4	0.8	0.8	80	10	200
40	0.2	13	1.1	1.0	1.0	4	0.9	0.9	100	10	250
40	0.3	15	1.2	1.1	1.2	5	1.0	1.0	110	10	250
40	0.4	17	1.3	1.3	1.4	5	1.2	1.2	125	10	300
45	0.4	18	1.4	1.4	1.6	5	1.4	1.4	135	18	350
55	0.4	20	1.5	1.5	1.8	5	1.4	1.4	150	18	400
60	0.4	18	16	1.4	2.0	5	0.8	0.8	140	10	400
60	0.4	18	1.7	1.4	2.0	5	0.8	0.8	140	10	350
60	0.4	17	1.7	1.3	2.0	5	0.8	0.8	125	10	350
60	0.4	14	1.7	1.2	2.0	6	0.8	0.8	110	10	350
40	0.4	15	1.3	1.1	1.4	5	1.2	1.2	110	18	300
45	0.4	15	1.4	1.2	1.6	5	1.3	1.3	115	18	350
50	0.4	16	1.4	1.2	1.8	5	1.3	1.3	120	18	350
50	0.4	15	1.5	1.2	2.0	5	1.3	1.3	115	18	350
50	0.4	15	1.5	1.2	2.0	5	1.3	1.3	115	18	350
55	0.4	13	1.5	1.0	2.0	5	0.8	0.8	100	18	300
55	0.4	13	1.5	1.0	2.0	5	0.8	0.8	90	18	300
55	0.4	13	1.5	1.0	2.0	6	0.8	0.8	80	10	300
60	0.8	15	1.8	+0.1	2.5	8	+0.4	+0.4	125	18	450
60	0.5	20	2.0	+0.5	2.5	6	+0.5	+0.5	150	18	450

3. The folacin allowances refer to dietary sources as determined by Lactobacillus casei assay. Pure forms of folacin may be effective in doses less than 1/4 of the RDA.

4. Niacin equivalents include dietary sources of the vitamin itself plus 1 mg equivalent for each 60 mg of dietary tryptophan.

5. Assumes protein equivalent to human milk. For proteins not 100 percent utilized factors should be increased proportionately.

Table reproduced with permission of the National Academy of Sciences.

Principal
References

PRINCIPAL REFERENCES

General

1. Altman, P. L. and Dittmer, D. S. (Eds.), *Biology Data Book*, Fed. Am. Soc. Exp. Biol., Washington, D.C. (1964).
2. Altman, P. L. and Dittmer, D. S. (Eds.), *Blood and Other Body Fluids*, Fed. Am. Soc. Exp. Biol., Washington, D.C. (1961).
3. Altman, P. L. and Dittmer, D. S. (Eds.), *Growth*, Fed. Am. Soc. Exp. Biol., Washington, D.C. (1962).
4. Altman, P. L. and Dittmer, D. S. (Eds.), *Metabolism*, Fed. Am. Soc. Exp. Biol., Washington, D.C. (1968).
5. Boyer, P. D. and Snell, E. E. (Eds.), *Annual Reviews of Biochemistry*, Vols. 36–39, Annual Reviews, Inc., Palo Alto, Calif. (1967–70).
6. Conn, E. E. and Stumpf, P. K., *Outlines of Biochemistry*, 2nd Ed., Wiley, New York (1966).
7. Dawson, R. M. C., Elliott, D. C., Elliot, W. H., and Jones, K. M. (Eds.), *Data for Biochemical Research*, 2nd Ed., Oxford Univ. Press. New York and Oxford (1969).
8. Diem, K. (Ed.), *Documenta Geigy Scientific Tables,* 6th Ed., Geigy Pharmaceuticals, Ardsley, N.Y. (1962).
9. Goodman, L. S. and Gilman, A. (Ed.), *The Pharmaceutical Basis of Therapeutics*, 4th Ed., Macmillan, New York (1970).
10. Greenberg, D. M. (Ed.), *Metabolic Pathways*, 3rd Ed., Vols. I–IV, Academic Press, New York and London (1967).
11. Harris, R. S., Wool, I. G., and Loraine, J. A. (Eds.) *Vitamins and Hormones*, Vols. 25–27, Academic Press, New York and London (1967–69).
12. Long, C. (Ed.), *Biochemists' Handbook*, Van Nostrand Reinhold, New York (1961).
13. Needham, A. E., *The Growth Process in Animals*, Van Nostrand Reinhold, New York (1964).

14. Oser, B. L. (Ed.), *Hawk's Physiological Chemistry*, 14th Ed., McGraw-Hill (Blakiston Div.), New York (1965).
15. Stecher, P. G. (Ed.), *The Merck Index*, 8th Ed., Merck & Co., Inc., Rahway, N.J. (1968).
16. Weast, R. C. (Ed.), *Handbook of Chemistry and Physics*, 49th Ed., The Chemical Rubber Co., Cleveland, Ohio (1968).
17. West, E. S., Todd, W. R., Mason, H. S., and Van Bruggen, J. T., *Textbook of Biochemistry*, 4th Ed., Macmillan, New York (1966).
18. Williams, R. J. and Lansford, E. M., Jr. (Eds.), *The Encyclopedia of Biochemistry*, Van Nostrand Reinhold, New York (1967).
19. *National Formulary*, XIII Ed., Prepared by National Formulary Board, Am. Pharmaceutical Assoc., Washington, D.C. (1970).
20. *The Pharmacopeia of the United States of America*, 18th Revision, Prepared by the Committee of Revision, The United States Pharmacopeial Convention, Inc., Bethesda, Md. (1971).

Specific: Vitamins

21. Bonner, J. and Varner, J. E. (Eds.), *Plant Biochemistry*, Academic Press, New York and London (1965).
22. Burton, B. T., *The Heinz Handbook of Nutrition*, 2nd Ed., H. J. Heinz Co. (McGraw-Hill), New York (1965).
23. Davidson, S. and Passmore, R., *Human Nutrition and Dietetics*, 4th Ed., Williams & Wilkins, Baltimore, Md. (1969).
24. DeLuca, H. F. and Suttie, J. W. (Eds.), *The Fat-Soluble Vitamins*, Univ. of Wisconsin Press, Madison, Wis. (1970).
25. Furia, T. E. (Ed.), *Handbook of Food Additives*, The Chemical Rubber Co., Cleveland, Ohio (1968).
26. Goodhart, R. S. and Wohl, M. G., *Manual of Clinical Nutrition*, Lea & Febiger, Philadelphia (1964).
27. Goodwin, T. W., *The Biosynthesis of Vitamins and Related Compounds*, Academic Press, London and New York (1963).
28. McCormick, D. B. and Wright, L. D. (Eds.), *Methods in Enzymology*, Vol. XVIII, *Vitamins and Coenzymes*, Parts A–C, Academic Press, New York and London (1970).
29. Morton, R. A. (Ed.), *Fat-Soluble Vitamins*, Pergamon Press, New York (1970).
30. Robinson, F. A., *The Vitamin Co-factors of Enzyme Systems*, Pergamon Press, New York (1966).
31. Rodale, J. I. and Staff, *The Complete Book of Vitamins*, Rodale Books, Inc., Emmaus, Pa. (1971).
32. Sebrell, W. H., Jr., and Harris, R. S. (Eds. Vols. I–V), Gyorgy, P. and Pearson, W. N. (Eds. Vols. VI–VII), *The Vitamins*, 2nd Ed., Vols. I–VII, Academic Press, New York and London (1967).
33. Strohecker, R. and Henning, H. M., *Vitamin Assay Tested Methods*, The Chemical Rubber Co., Cleveland, Ohio (1966).
34. Wagner, A. F. and Folkers, K., *Vitamins and Coenzymes*, Wiley (Interscience Div.), New York (1964).
35. Wohl, M. G. and Goodhart, R. S. (Eds.), *Modern Nutrition in Health and Disease*, 4th Ed., Lea & Febiger, Philadelphia (1968).
36. National Research Council Pub. #1694, *Recommended Dietary Allowances*, 7th Revised Ed., Printing and Publishing Office, National Academy of Sciences, Washington, D.C. (1968).

Specific: Hormones

37. Back, N., Martini, L. and Paoletti, R. (Eds.), "Pharmacology of Hormonal Polypeptides and Proteins" in *Advances in Exp. Med. Biol.,* Vol. 2, Plenum Press, New York (1968).
38. Briggs, M. H. (Ed.), *Advances in Steroid Biochemistry and Pharmacology*, Vols. 1 and 2, Academic Press, New York and London (1970).
39. Briggs, M. H. and Brotherton, J., *Steroid Biochemistry and Pharmacology*, Academic Press, London and New York (1970).
40. Butt, W. R., *Hormone Chemistry*, Van Nostrand Reinhold, New York (1967).
41. Eisenstein, A. B. (Ed.), *The Adrenal Cortex*, Little, Brown and Co., Boston (1967).
42. Fieser, L. F. and Fieser, M., *Steroids*, Van Nostrand Reinhold, New York (1959).
43. Frieden, E. and Lipner, H., *Biochemical Endocrinology of the Vertebrates*, Prentice-Hall, Englewood Cliffs, N.J. (1971).
44. Gray, C. H. and Bacharach, A. L. (Eds.), *Hormones in Blood*, 2nd Ed., Vols. 1 and 2, Academic Press, London and New York (1967).
45. Heftmann, E. and Mosettig, E., *Biochemistry of Steroids*, Van Nostrand Reinhold, New York (1960).
46. Krüskemper, H. L., *Anabolic Steroids*, Academic Press, New York and London (1968).
47. Litwack, G. (Ed.), *Biochemical Actions*, Vols. I and II, Academic Press, New York and London (1970).
48. Martini, L. and Ganong, W. F. (Eds.), *Neuroendocrinology*, Vols. I and II, Academic Press, New York and London (1967).
49. McKerns, K. W., *Steroid Hormones and Metabolism*, Appleton-Century-Crofts (Meredith Corp.), New York (1969).
50. Sawin, C. T., *The Hormones*, Little, Brown and Co., Boston (1969).
51. Stear, E. B., and Kadish, A. H. (Eds.), *Hormonal Control Systems*, Elsevier, New York (1969).
52. Tepperman, J., *Metabolic and Endocrine Physiology*, 2nd Ed., Year Book Medical Publishers, Chicago (1968).
53. Turner, C. D. and Bagnara, J. T., *General Endocrinology*, 5th Ed., Saunders, Philadelphia (1971).
54. Von Euler, U. S. and Heller, H. (Eds.), *Comparative Endocrinology*, Vols. I and II, Academic Press, New York and London (1963).
55. Williams, R. H. (Ed.), *Textbook of Endocrinology*, 4th Ed., Saunders, Phildelphia (1968).
56. Zarrow, M. X., Yochim, J. M. and McCarthy, J. L., *Experimental Endocrinology*, Academic Press, New York and London (1964).

ITEMIZED TABLE OF REFERENCES[a]

	Vitamins	Hormones
GENERAL INFORMATION		
1. Synonyms	7, 15, 17, 34	1, 7, 15
2. History	15, 17, 18, 34	9, 15, 18, 42, 52
3. Physiological Forms	17, 25 32	9, 44, 55
4. Active Analogs	14, 17, 25, 32	40, 42, 55
5. Inactive Analogs	14, 17, 32	38, 39, 40, 42, 55
6. Antagonists	1, 7, 14, 17, 32	9, 17, 40
7. Synergists	1, 7, 14, 17, 32	9, 17, 40
8. Physiological Functions	4, 14, 22, 32	3, 4, 8, 17, 41, 55
9. Deficiency Diseases	4, 14, 17, 32	3, 14, 17, 55
10. Essentiality	1, 4, 14, 32	1, 9, 53
CHEMISTRY		
1. Structure	1, 8, 16, 17, 24, 29, 30, 32, 34	1, 8, 9, 15, 16, 45
2. Reactions	4, 15, 17, 20, 24, 29, 30, 32, 34	1, 8, 9, 15, 20
3. Properties	1, 7, 15, 16, 19, 24, 29, 30, 32	1, 7, 8, 9, 15, 16, 19, 20, 37
4. Commercial Production	15, 24, 29, 30, 32, 34	9, 15, 40, 42
5. Isolation	9, 24, 29, 30, 32, 34,	40, 42
6. Determination	14, 17, 33	1, 14, 40, 44, 53, 56
DISTRIBUTION AND SOURCES		
1. Occurrence	17, 22, 24, 27, 29, 30, 32, 34	
2. Dietary Sources	4, 8, 12, 22, 24, 27, 29, 30, 32	
MEDICAL AND BIOLOGICAL ROLE		
1. Species	—	1, 53, 54
2. Units	8, 17, 32	8, 9, 14
3. Blood Levels	2, 8, 14, 32	2, 8, 14
4. Requirements	4, 8, 23, 26, 31, 36	—
5. Administration	8, 9, 30, 34	8, 9, 38, 55
6. Factors Affecting Availability or Release	4, 8, 22, 31	1, 3, 4, 50
7. Deficiency	4, 17, 23, 26, 31, 35	1, 3, 4, 53, 55
8. Overdose	4, 17, 24, 29, 30, 32	1, 3, 4, 38, 53, 55
METABOLIC ROLE		
1. Biosynthesis and Production Sites	4, 21, 27, 28	38, 39, 40, 41, 55
2. Storage Areas	8, 9, 17, 32	8, 9, 17

[a] Numbers under Vitamin and Hormone columns refer to those in list of principal references.

ITEMIZED TABLE OF REFERENCES (*cont.*)

	Vitamins	Hormones
METABOLIC ROLE (*cont.*)		
3. Blood Carriers	2, 8, 14, 29, 30	2, 8, 40, 44
4. Half-life	8, 9, 29, 30, 32	8, 9, 44
5. Target Tissues	14, 17, 29, 30, 32	1, 3, 38, 40
6. Reactions	5, 14, 17, 28	4, 5, 40, 43, 46, 49, 50, 53
7. Mode of Action	4, 5, 6, 9, 14, 22, 24	3, 4, 5, 8, 9, 17, 47, 51, 55
8. Catabolism	1, 8, 9, 10, 17, 28	1, 9, 40, 43, 49, 50
MISCELLANEOUS		
1. (Other) Vitamins	8, 11, 13, 30	8, 11, 13, 53
2. (Other) Hormones	8, 11, 13, 53	8, 11, 13, 48, 53
3. Unusual Properties	11, 13, 14, 17	46, 48, 53
4. Relationships	11, 13, 38	11, 13, 38

Index

(Entries followed by T denote Tables)